Biopsy Diagnosis
in
Rheumatic Diseases

Biopsy Diagnosis
in
Rheumatic Diseases

J. T. Lie
MD, MS, FACC, FACA, FACR, FCCP
Formerly Professor of Pathology, Mayo Medical School
and Mayo Graduate School of Medicine
Consultant in Pathology, Cardiovascular Diseases and Internal Medicine,
Mayo Clinic and Mayo Foundation
Rochester, Minnesota

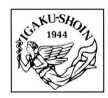

IGAKU-SHOIN   New York • Tokyo

Cover Illustration: Plexogenic pulmonary hypertension in rheumatic diseases.

Published and distributed by

IGAKU-SHOIN Medical Publishers, Inc.
One Madison Avenue, New York, New York 10010

IGAKU-SHOIN Ltd.,
5-24-3 Hongo, Bunkyo-ku, Tokyo 113-91

Library of Congress Cataloging-in-Publication Data

Lie, J. T.
    Biopsy diagnosis in rheumatic diseases / J.T. Lie.
        p.   cm.
    Includes bibliographical references and index.
    ISBN 0-89640-327-0. — ISBN 4-260-14327-1
    1. Connective tissue—Diseases—Histopathology.   2. Connective
tissue—Biopsy   3. Rheumatism—Histopathology.   I. Title.
    [DNLM: 1. Rheumatic Diseases—pathology.   2. Biopsy—methods.   WE
544L716b 1997]
RC924.L54 1997
616.7'2307583—dc20
DNLM/DLC
for Library of Congress   96-29142
                                                                          CIP

ISBN: 0-89640-327-0   (New York)
ISBN: 4-260-14327-1   (Tokyo)

Printed and bound in the U.S.A.
10 9 8 7 6 5 4 3 2 1

Dedication

To

Dr. Margaret Ruth Macfarlane Lie

My wife and best friend, who is also
the ideal mother and a role model physician-physiatrist

Foreword – 1

It is a pleasure to write this foreword to Dr. J. T. Lie's excellent volume on *Biopsy Diagnosis in Rheumatic Diseases*. The definition of histologic alterations of the involved tissues is an integral part in the description of human disease. An understanding of these changes is requisite for the physician who wants to understand the nature of the pathologic processes. Such histopathologic findings in affected body parts form a base which can be used to guide care of the patient and also provide insights to further study or research regarding a disease. The histopathology of most rheumatic diseases may not always be specifically distinctive to be pathognomonic in itself, but when correlated with clinical findings it provides enough information to sufficiently confirm or document the diagnosis. Advances in molecular biology have provided new tools to elucidate the heretofore ill-understood pathogenesis of many rheumatic disorders but histopathology will continue to be an essential component in the diagnosis, treatment, and clinical investigation of rheumatic diseases in the future.

In my training and early years as a practitioner, I often went with our house staff to the operating room to watch an operation on one of our patients, and we would later visit the pathology laboratory to review the biopsy with a pathologist. As medical practice becomes more complex and demanding, there is less time and opportunity and more impediments to visiting the operating suite and the pathology laboratory. Dr. Lie's book will help counteract or fill the gap in this emerging deficit in our training and practice. The book provides an authoritative source for illustrative histopathology found in the various inflammatory rheumatic diseases for the student, physician (especially the rheumatologist), and less experienced or unspecialized pathologist. Dr. Lie is an exacting scholar and thoughtful teacher who has developed a vast experience in the pathology of rheumatic diseases. His perspective is broad and balanced; and he never fails to emphasize the importance of clinicopathologic correlation. A perusal of Dr. Lie's book is the next best thing to actually reviewing the histology slides with an expert tutor.

Gene G. Hunder, MD, FACP, FACR
Chair, Division of Rheumatology
Mayo Clinic and Mayo Medical School
Rochester, Minnesota

Foreword – 2

The many connective tissue or rheumatic disorders differ in their clinical manifestations, immunologic abnormalities, types of tissue changes, and undoubtedly, in their etiology and pathogenesis. While diseases of practically every organ of the body are dealt with in a comprehensive manner in standard large textbooks, there are also shorter, specialty books that describe the pathologic changes of diseases and correlate them with the clinical data in order to provide clues to diagnosis, prognosis, and therapy. The present book belongs to the latter and very useful category. It does not attempt to explore the etiology and pathogenesis of rheumatic diseases, many of which are expressions of autoimmunity and account for their serologic manifestations discussed in detail in larger textbooks.

Dr. J. T. Lie is eminently qualified to author this book. It is based on his extensive experience with rheumatic diseases at the Mayo Clinic and elsewhere. The descriptions and the comments are succinct and clearly presented, making it readily accessible to the interested clinicians and pathologists. The illustrations, drawn from his own vast collection, are of the highest quality. He is also the sole author, thus providing a consistent point of view and avoiding duplications.

The inclusion of entities that are not truly classic rheumatic diseases, but are often seen by the rheumatologists, broadens the scope of the book and assists in differential diagnosis. All disease entities are described in sufficient detail to furnish the reader with up-to-date information. Historical introduction in each chapter adds up to a brief history of rheumatic diseases, and provides a better understanding of their mutual relationship. Advice about tissue processing and staining of biopsies will help the pathologist to have adequate slides for evaluation, while suggestions about the best sites or tissues for biopsy will assist the clinician in obtaining optimal material for diagnosis.

The book is highly recommended to anyone interested in the diagnosis of rheumatic diseases.

Jacob Churg, MD
Professor Emeritus of Pathology
Mount Sinai School of Medicine
New York, New York

Acknowledgments

This book could not have been written and published without the goodwill and assistance of many people. I am singularly indebted to the generous referral of clinical materials from the clinicians and pathologists at home and abroad; although too numerous to be mentioned individually, my gratitude is no less sincere.

The following illustrations are reproduced with permission:

Figure 3.5, from Dr. Xavier Puéchal of Paris
Figure 5.4, from Dr. Edenilson Eduardo Calore of Sào Paulo
Figure 7.12 and 8.6, from Dr. Jacob Churg of New York
Figure 13.1, from Dr. Kevin Davies of London

Some of the author's own previously published illustrations are reproduced with permissions, while others are reproduced by virtue of retained copyright ownership.

Special thanks are due Dr. Gene Hunder and Dr. Jacob Churg for their encouragement and for their gracious *Forewords,* written from the perspective of a rheumatologist and a pathologist, respectively; Lila Maron, Vice President, Editorial, Igaku-Shoin Medical Publishers, New York, for facilitating the acquisition negotiation and arrangement to have the book published within six months of complete manuscript submission; Sherri Souffrance, Production Director, for her care, patience, and expert advice in every phase of the production of this book; and Dr. Margaret Lie for undertaking the tedious, repetitive, and exacting chore of proof-reading the manuscript, truly a labor of love.

Preface

Arthritis and other rheumatic diseases afflict many and are common severely disabling health care problems. The prevalence rate of self-reported arthritis and other rheumatic diseases in the United States is projected to increase from 15.0% (37.9 million) of the 1990 population to 18.2% (59.4 million) of the estimated 2020 population.

The term "rheumatic diseases" encompasses a large family of etiologically different categories of diverse clinical entities, numbering in excess of two hundreds, of which the most important are the classic connective tissue diseases. The diagnosis of most rheumatic diseases is usually based on clinical and serological findings, supplemented by other selective laboratory tests and radiologic imaging techniques. However, in many instances, a definitive diagnosis is not possible without the appropriate biopsy confirmation. A diagnostic manual on the histopathology of those rheumatic diseases and related disorders that lend themselves to biopsy procedures would be highly desirable for the clinician and pathologist alike, but one does not exist, and this book is an attempt to fill that void.

This book on biopsy diagnosis is based on the author's career-long interest in the pathology of rheumatic diseases and related disorders. This interest began in 1969 when the author first became associated with the Mayo Clinic in Rochester, Minnesota, where the work of Philip S. Hench and Edward C. Kendall on the treatment of rheumatic diseases with cortisone earned them the 1950 Nobel Prize in Physiology and Medicine. Having the good fortune of developing one's career in academic medicine at an institution steeped in the tradition of excellent patient-care, and working closely with a large group of dedicated clinical rheumatologists, have nurtured, fortified, and sustained the author's interest in the pathology of rheumatic diseases, and the desire to share this experience with others.

The clinical entities discussed in this book include the major classic connective tissue diseases as well as clinical syndromes that are not strictly or traditionally rheumatic in nature but the practicing rheumatologists nevertheless have also been frequently called upon to manage patients with these systemic disorders. Each entity discussed in this book is introduced with a synoptic description from the broad historical and clinical perspectives to provide a more sure footing for a rational approach to the biopsy diagnosis of rheumatic diseases, its value and limitations. The variety and details of biopsies described, and illustrated, obviously would vary according to the individual entities; the discussion on some entities are more limited than that of others because of the differences in their accessibility to biopsy, but a balanced presentation is intended and attempted where possible. Biopsy diagnosis of rheumatic diseases in the subspecialties of neuropathology (for neuromuscular disorders), orthopedic pathology (for bone, cartilage, and joint disorders), and renal pathology (for renal parenchymal disorders), is outside the purview and scope of this book.

The format of books in the Igaku-Shoin's Series on *Differential Diagnosis in Pathology* is ideal for the presentation of a reader-friendly and practical diagnostic manual, and a similar format is adopted here. The text is uncluttered with punctuated reference citations, and there is no contrived compulsion to justify every statement made and every number given. For those who desire further reading or wish to consult the original source of the information, pertinent key references for each chapter are grouped together as the *Bibliography*. In addition to the important historical accounts and selected classic articles of interest, regardless of their years of publication, as much current literature published in the 1990s, as it is available to press time, has been cited. The liberal inclusion of illustrations is another basic necessity and appeal that all useful manuals of diagnostic pathology must have. The overall layout and the text:figures ratios in different chapters are determined by the unique nature and individuality of the topics under discussion.

It is hoped that the practicing general and specialist pathologists and pathology trainees; rheumatologists and rheumatology trainees; general physicians and clinical investigators; residents and senior medical students, will find this a useful reference manual on the biopsy diagnosis of rheumatic diseases. We should all be reminded of the importance of thoughtful clinicopathologic correlations in the interpretation of biopsy findings, applicable to rheumatic disorders as much as it is to other diseases.

Contents

Section 1 INTRODUCTION

1. Nomenclature, Classification, and Biopsy Diagnosis in Rheumatic Diseases

NOMENCLATURE

'What's in a name?' Shakespeare W. *Romeo and Juliet.* Act II; scene 2; line 43.

Arthritis and rheumatism, diffuse connective tissue disease, diffuse collagen disease, or *diffuse vascular disease,* known by any other name, rheumatic diseases are maladies of antiquity dating back to the time of Hippocrates of Cos (c. 460 to c. 375 B.C.).

The term *rheum* or *rheuma* (meaning "flux" or "catarrhal discharge") belongs to the ancient theory of disease and is encountered in the 4th century B.C. in the portion of the Hippocratic corpus entitled *On the Location in the Human Body.* The concept of rheumatism as a systemic disease was probably introduced in the seventeenth century by the Parisian physician Guillaume Baillou (Ballonius) (1558–1616) in a posthumously published work, in 1642, entitled *The Book on Rheumatism and Back Pain,* in which he pronounced "what arthritis is in a joint that is exactly what rheumatism is in the body." In Dunglison's 1874 dictionary of medical science, *rheumatism* was defined as "a kind of shifting phlegmasia or neuralgia, sometimes seated in the muscles, sometimes in the parts surrounding the joints; and at others, within them." William Heberden, of the angina pectoris fame, foresaw the potential problem of nomenclature and classification of rheumatic diseases when he commented, in 1802, "The rheumatism is a common name for many aches and pains, which have yet got no peculiar appellation, though owing to very different causes. It is besides often hard to be distinguished from some, which have a certain name and class assigned them."

The German pathologist, Fritz Klinge, credited the French physician and founder of histology, Marie François Xavier Bichat (1771–1802) with introducing the idea, in 1801, that rheumatic diseases primarily affect the fibrous tissue of the body. Klinge himself, in 1933 and 1934, also conceived the notion that the characteristic organ and tissue alterations in rheumatic fever and rheumatoid arthritis reflect a systemic involvement of the entire connective tissues of the human body.

The term *diffuse vascular disease* was used by the Boston physician Benjamin Bank, in 1941, to include scleroderma, dermatomyositis, disseminated lupus erythematosus, and polyarteritis nodosa, on the basis that "all of which represent a widespread vascular involvement, differing usually in the extent of the pathologic change, the size of the vessels involved, and the organs chiefly affected." Three physicians working at the Mount Sinai Hospital in New York, Paul Klemperer, Abou Pollack, and George Baehr, in 1942, proposed that since both systemic lupus erythematosus and scleroderma were characterized microscopically by "fundamental alteration of the collagenous tissues" they could be viewed as "systemic diseases of the connective tissue." They expressed this concept by the name *diffuse collagen disease,* a metaphor in which *collagen* stood for connective tissue in its entirety. The term was used "because of the conspicuous morbid manifestations of the extracellular components," not because it was believed that these diseases specially affected the substance collagen. The hybrid name *collagen-vascular disease* was introduced, in 1946, by the pathologist Arnold Rich at the Johns Hopkins Hospital to unify the two views (*collagen* and *vascular* involvement) of the pathology of "a group of diseases that are highly important because of their incapacitating or lethal potentials," including polyarteritis nodosa, rheumatic fever, systemic lupus erythematosus, and rheumatoid arthritis. Neither the clinical features nor the histopathological changes of rheumatic diseases defines a homogeneous and distinctive group of disorders, and this prompted Klemperer's prediction, in 1950, that *collagen disease* "may become a catch-all term for maladies with puzzling clinical and anatomical features," which it has.

CLASSIFICATION

". . . any classification is necessarily incomplete and acts as a bridge between complete ignorance and total understanding." Goodwin JF. *Br Heart J* 1982;48: 1–18

Each patient with a rheumatic disease may be unique, and the rheumatologist needs to communicate with others when referring to different groups of patients sharing similar clinical signs, symptoms, and prognosis, which necessitates specific diagnoses and a classification of rheumatic diseases.

A classification should ideally be based on the etiology and pathogenesis of diseases but this is not possible because most rheumatic diseases are clinical entities of unknown cause. The two attempts by the American

Table 1.1 Ten Major Categories in the 1983 American Rheumatism Association Nomenclature and Classification of Rheumatic Diseases*

I.	Diffuse connective tissue diseases
II.	Arthritis associated with spondylitis
III.	Osteoarthritis and degenerative joint disease
IV.	Rheumatic disorders associated with infectious agents
V.	Rheumatic disorders associated with metabolic and endocrine diseases
VI.	Neoplastic diseases
VII.	Neurovascular disorders
VIII.	Bone and cartilage disorders
IX.	Extraarticular disorders
X.	Miscellaneous disorders associated with articular manifestations

*Adapted from Decker et al. *Arthritis Rheum* 26: 1029–1032, 1983.

Rheumatism Association (now the American College of Rheumatology), in 1964 and 1983, to classify rheumatic diseases resulted in a compilation and grouping of individual entities by categories; the 1964 classification listed more than 100 kinds of "arthritis" and the 1983 classification inventoried more than 200 conditions and syndromes in 10 major categories (Table 1). The 1983 Glossary Subcommittee of the American Rheumatism Association Committee on Rheumatologic Practice rightfully justified its approach to classification with the following statement: "A classification is primarily a record of the insights achieved to date. The inevitable constraint it imposes acts to make the unusual stand out, thereby providing the potential for new insights, greater knowledge, and future classification." This 1983 all-inclusive umbrella classification of rheumatic diseases has been supplemented and complemented by a series of *Classification Criteria* for a number of individual entities, such as: rheumatic fever, rheumatoid arthritis, osteoarthritis, gout, systemic lupus erythematosus, systemic sclerosis (scleroderma), vasculitis, and fibromyalgia, many of which are undergoing periodic revisions, and the list of entities is growing.

The clinical entities discussed in this book include most of the classic diffuse connective tissue diseases and selected diseases and syndromes which may not be traditional or strictly rheumatic in nature but the practicing rheumatologists nevertheless have also been frequently called upon to manage patients with these systemic disorders, listed in the *Table of Contents.*

BIOPSY DIAGNOSIS OF RHEUMATIC DISEASES

"It is necessary not only to have satisfactory biopsy specimens, but it is particularly important to have an interested and experienced pathologist who is willing to glean everything possible from these tiny pieces of tissue. If such a person is not available, the endoscopist need not attempt transbronchoscopic lung biopsies." Anderson HA   *Chest* 1978;73:734–736.

The diagnosis of most of the common and uncommon rheumatic diseases is essentially clinical and serological, incorporating additional relevant laboratory tests and current radiologic imaging techniques. However, a definitive diagnosis is not possible without biopsy confirmation in many instances, and there are also rheumatic diseases that do not lend themselves to biopsy diagnosis. Biopsy is a valuable diagnostic tool applicable to most of the "diffuse connective tissue diseases" category of the 1983 American Rheumatism Association Classification of Arthritis and Rheumatism (Table 1.1). Excluded for discussion in this book are those categories identified with infectious diseases; degenerative, metabolic, and endocrine disorders; neoplasms; primary and hereditary neuromuscular diseases; bone and cartilage disorders; extra-articular and miscellaneous disorders; which fall under, more appropriately, the purview of their respective subspecialties, such as neuropathology, orthopedic pathology, and renal pathology.

Because rheumatic diseases are after all, "collagen-vascular diseases," all histologic materials processed for light microscopy should be routinely prepared with, in addition to the usual hematoxylin-eosin, stains for elastin and fibrous connective tissue (often combined as a single "elastic-trichrome" stain). Other special stains may be added as needed, to identify or confirm the presence of, for instance, amyloid, acid mucopolysaccharides, α-1-antitrypsin, calcium, iron, and mast cells. The interpretation of biopsies in rheumatic diseases is subject to such variables as the examining pathologist's expertise, tissue selection, sample size, chronologic age of the disease process and any prior treatment at the time of biopsy; whether serial or step-sections are prepared; and, most of all, clinicopathologic correlation. A biopsy is adequate only when it provides a verifiable diagnosis; and a negative biopsy cannot always exclude a disease in question with focal lesions. It is always helpful to discuss the biopsy findings of complicated or indeterminate types of cases with the attending physician and/or radiologist to exchange information and to express the degree of confidence of the biopsy diagnosis.

BIBLIOGRAPHY

Banks BM: Is there a common denominator in scleroderma, dermatomyositis, disseminated lupus erythematosus, the Libman-Sacks syndrome and polyarteritis nodosa? *N Engl J Med* 255:433–444, 1941.

Benedek TG, Rodnan GP: A brief history of the rheumatic diseases. *Bull Rheum Dis* 32:59–68, 1982.

Blumberg BS, Bunim JJ, Calkins E, Pirani CL, Zvaifler NJ: Nomenclature and classification of arthritis and rheumatism (tentative) accepted by the American Rheumatism Association. *Bull Rheum Dis* 14:339–340, 1964.

Bywaters EGL: The historical evolution of the concept of connective tissue diseases. *Scand J Rheumatol* 5:11–29, 1976.

Decker JL and the Glossary Subcommittee of the ARA Committee on Rheumatologic Practice: American Rheumatism Association nomenclature and classification of arthritis and rheumatism (1983). *Arthritis Rheum* 26:1029–1032, 1983.

Heberden W: *Commentaries on the History and Cure of Diseases.* London, T Payne, 1802:397.

Favus MJ (ed): *Primer on the metabolic bone disease and disorders of mineral metabolism,* ed 2. Philadelphia, Lippincott-Raven publishers, 1993, 441 pp.

Fries JF, Hochberg MC, Medsger TA, Jr, et al: Criteria for rheumatic disease: Different types and different functions. *Arthritis Rheum* 37:454–462, 1994.

Gardner DL: *Pathological Basis of the Connective Tissue Disease.* London, Lea & Febiger, 1992, 1050pp.

Grishman E, Churg J, Needle MA, Venkataseshan VS (eds): *The Kidney in Collagen-Vascular Diseases.* New York, Raven Press, 1993, 258pp.

Klemperer P, Pollack AD, Baehr G: Diffuse collagen disease: Acute disseminated lupus erythematosus and diffuse scleroderma. *JAMA* 119:331–332, 1942.

Klemperer P: The concept of collagen diseases. *Am J Pathol* 26:505–519, 1950.

Klinge F: Der "Rheumatismus"-begriff in geschichtlicher Betrachtung. *Jahresk Aerztl Fortbild* 24:1–16, 1933.

Klinge F: Zur Pathologischen Anatomie des Rheumatismus. *Verh Dtsch Orthop Ges* 28:44–50, 1934.

Lie JT: Recognizing coronary heart disease: Selected historical vignettes from the period of William Harvey (1578–1657) to Adam Hammar (1818–1878). *Mayo Clin Proc* 53:811–817, 1978.

Parish LC: An historical approach to the nomenclature of rheumatoid arthritis. *Arthritis Rheum* 6:138–158, 1963.

Reynolds MD: Origin of the concept of Collagen-vascular diseases. *Semin Arthritis Rheum* 15:127–131, 1985.

Schumacher HR, Klippel JH, Koopman WJ (eds): *Primer on the Rheumatic Diseases,* ed 10. Atlanta, The Arthritis Foundation, 1993, 347 pp.

von Mühlen CA, Tan EM: Autoantibodies in the diagnosis of systemic rheumatic diseases. *Semin Arthritis Rheum* 24:323–358, 1995.

Section 2

CLASSIC CONNECTIVE TISSUE DISEASES

2. Rheumatic Fever

In 1836, the French physician Jean-Baptisle Bouillaud (1796–1881) called attention to the relationship of acute generalized febrile articular rheumatism to disease of the heart, which might have been the first clinical description of rheumatic carditis as we now know it. In 1881, Jean-Martin Charcot (1825–1893) was probably referring to the sequelae of rheumatic carditis when he proclaimed, "I have collected a considerable number of cases in which endocarditis has developed in chronic rheumatism without the disease ever having assumed an acute form." The cause of rheumatic carditis became apparent some 50 years later.

Group A streptococcal infection is notorious for its association with two potentially serious, nonsuppurative sequelae: acute rheumatic fever (ARF) and poststreptococcal acute glomerulonephritis (PSAGN). These two poststreptococcal disorders are immunologically mediated but the mechanisms responsible for each are likely to be distinct; the two organs affected in ARF and PSAGN are not directly invaded by the microorganisms.

The dramatic decline in incidence of ARF in the United States during the past half century has been a truly remarkable phenomenon: from an incidence rate of 388 per 100,000 among army personnel in the 1940s, to 25–35 per 100,000 among school children in the 1960s, to an overall rate of 0.5–1.88 per 100,000 in the 1980s. A new, equally surprising and highly disturbing change in the epidemiology of ARF may be in the making, beginning in the mid-1980s, with reports from several U.S. cities suggesting a resurgence of ARF in this country. Just as the dramatic decline remains unexplained, so does the resurgence. Of interest, the preceding pharyngitis has been mild in the majority of cases but the incidence of carditis has been high (>90% in one series), and the ARF has been concentrated in middle class families with ready access to medical care. Even more intriguing has been the emergence of very mucoid strains of group A streptococci at the same time, but no "rheumatogenic factor" has yet been isolated from these strains. The Jones Criteria for guidance in clinical and laboratory diagnosis of ARF, initially proposed in 1944, has been modified, revised, and updated in 1992.

RHEUMATIC CARDITIS

Carditis is a major morphologic criterion for the diagnosis of ARF. Clinical evidence of carditis includes heart murmurs, cardiomegaly, pericarditis, and congestive heart failure. Pathologically, cardiac manifestations of ARF may include pericarditis, myocarditis, and endocarditis, or, various combinations of the three, but all of which may be nonspecific. The German pathologist, Ludwig Aschoff (1866–1942), first described a diagnostic lesion in the heart of ARF in 1904, later to become known as *Aschoff bodies* (or nodules), which are unique granulomatous lesions of controversial histogenesis. Lack of Aschoff body labeling for desmin and muscle-specific actin, S-100 and neurofilament, and *Ulex europeus* I and Factor VIII-related antigen is against derivation from vascular smooth muscle or cardiac myocyte, nerve or nerve sheath, and lymphatic or vascular endothelium, respectively. Strong labeling of Aschoff cells for vimentin is evidence for a mesenchymal origin, and labeling for myeloid cell or histiocyte antigen is consistent with a histiocytic origin.

Aschoff bodies in ARF-related carditis may be indefinitely persistent in the affected heart; they have been well documented in autopsy material and in cardiac tissue obtained at valve replacement surgery of patients with chronic rheumatic heart disease. In autopsy studies, the reported incidence of Aschoff bodies varies widely from 9 to 84% (average 42%); the incidence in surgical specimens (usually atrial appendages and papillary muscles) is just as variable, from 19 to 74% (average 38%). Although endomyocardial biopsy (EMB) became established as a safe diagnostic procedure in the early 1970s, mainly to monitor cardiac allograft rejection, diagnosis of acute rheumatic carditis by EMB was seldom carried out; it was first described by Ursell et al. in 1982 and there have been very few other similar reports. This is not surprising because until recently ARF was a vanishing disease in the developed countries worldwide, and rheumatic carditis is usually diagnosed clinically without biopsy confirmation. Among our referral cases of ARF biopsies there were 4 positive EMBs in 12 attempted biopsies: 2 had Aschoff bodies and 2 showed only myocarditis.

Although they superficially resemble each other, Aschoff bodies should not be confused with rheumatoid nodules; the former occur only in the heart while the latter are ubiquitous and, despite the name, they may be encountered in conditions other than rheumatoid arthritis.

The Aschoff body is considered pathognomonic of rheumatic carditis; being most characteristic and diagnostic in the so-called granulomatous stage, located principally in perivascular areas and subendocardial regions of the ventricular or atrial myocardium and,

9

rarely, in valvular tissue. An Aschoff body consists of myocardial histiocytes, the Anitschkow cells, fibroblasts, and lymphomononuclear cells arranged in rows or as clusters; a central core of fibrinoid necrosis may or may not be evident in an isolated histologic section (Figs. 2.1 and 2.2). The typical perivascular location of Aschoff bodies may not be demonstrable without examining serial sections (Fig. 2.3), and the so-called Aschoff giant cells are seen only rarely (Fig. 2.4). The endomyocardial infiltrate of Aschoff bodies consists of predominantly T-cells and occasionally B-cells. In one study of 50 surgical specimens, the relative percentages of T helper-inducer, T suppressor-cytotoxic lymphocytes, and macrophages, were 45.1 $\pm$ 7.6, 23.5 $\pm$ 4.8, and 29.3 $\pm$ 9.6%, respectively.

On the other hand, the myocarditis in ARF is non-specific; it may have predominantly a lymphoplasmacytic infiltrate, with or without discernible cardiac myocyte necrosis, or it may be granulomatous in character, the latter is morphologically indistinguishable from rheumatoid myocarditis (Figs. 2.5 and 2.6). Extracardiac involvement in ARF may include skin, muscle, synovium, lung, kidney, and the central nervous system, but they occur infrequently and the lesions are virtually never biopsied.

BIBLIOGRAPHY

Aschoff L: Zur Myocarditisfrage. *Verh Dtsch Ges Pathol* 8:46–53, 1904.

Benatar A, Beatty DW, Human DG: Immunological abnormalities in children with acute rheumatic carditis and acute poststreptococcal glomerulonephritis. *Int J Cardiol* 21:51–58, 1988.

Benedek TG: Subcutaneous nodules and the differentiation of rheumatoid arthritis from rheumatic fever. *Semin Arthritis Rheum* 13:305–321, 1984.

Bennett GA, Zeller JW, Bauer W: Subcutaneous nodules of rheumatoid arthritis and rheumatic fever. *Arch Pathol* 30:70–89, 1940.

Bisno AL, Shulman ST, Dajani AS: The rise and fall (and rise?) of rheumatic fever. *JAMA* 259:728–729, 1988.

Bisno AL: The coexistence of acute rheumatic fever and acute glomerulonephritis. *Arthritis Rheum* 32:230–232, 1989.

Bywaters EGL: The relation between heart and joint disease including "rheumatic heart disease" and chronic post-rheumatic arthritis (type Jaccoud). *Br Heart J* 12:101–131, 1950.

Chopra P: Origin of Ashoff nodule: An ultrastructural, light microscopic and histochemical evaluation. *Jpn Heart J* 25:227–235, 1985.

Chopra P, Narula J, Kumar AS, et al: Immunohistochemical characterisation of Aschoff nodules and endomyocardial inflammatory infiltrates in left atrial appendages from patients with chronic rheumatic heart disease. *Int J Cardiol* 20:99–105, 1988.

Council on Cardiovascular Disease in the Young of the American Heart Association: Guidelines for the diagnosis of rheumatic fever: Jones criteria, 1992 update. *JAMA* 268:2069–2073, 1992.

Dastur DK, Vevaina SC, Manghani DK, Shah NA: Changes in atrial biopsies in chronic rheumatic heart disease. 1. Cellulovascular and mesenchymal reaction. *Pathol Res Pract* 179:591–599, 1985.

Gardner DG: *Pathological Basis of the Connective Tissue Diseases.* Philadelphia, Lea & Febiger, 1992: 796–819.

Fassbender HG: *Pathology of Rheumatic Diseases.* (Translated by G. Loewi) New York, Springer-Verlag, 1975, pp 19–78.

Husby G, Arora R, Williams RC, et al: Immunofluorescence studies of florid rheumatic Aschoff lesions. *Arthritis Rheum* 29:207–211, 1986.

Kaplan EL, Markowitz M: The fall and rise of rheumatic fever in the United States: A commentary. *Int J Cardiol* 21:3–10, 1988.

Lie JT: Myocarditis and endomyocardial biopsy in unexplained heart failure: A diagnosis in search of a disease. *Ann Intern Med* 109:525–528, 1988.

Love GL, Restrepo C: Aschoff bodies of rheumatic carditis are granulomatous lesions of histocytic origin. *Modern Pathol* 1:256–261, 1988.

McKeown F: The pathology of rheumatic fever. *Ulster Med J* 14:97–107, 1945.

Persellin ST, Ramirez G, Moatamed F: Immunopathology of rheumatic pericarditis. *Arthritis Rheum* 25:1054–1058, 1982.

Roberts WC, Virmani R: Aschoff bodies at necropsy in valvular heart disease. *Circulation* 57:803–807, 1978.

Saphir O: The Aschoff nodule. *Am J Clin Pathol* 31:534–539, 1959.

Tedeschi CG, Wagner BM, Pani KC: Studies in rheumatic fever: I. The clinical significance of the Aschoff body based on morphologic observations. *Arch Pathol Lab Med* 60:408–422, 1955.

Ursell PC, Albala A, Fenoglio JJ: Diagnosis of acute rheumatic carditis by endomyocardial biopsy. *Hum Pathol* 13:677–679, 1982.

Vevaina SC, Dastur DK, Manghani DK, Shah NA: Changes in atrial biopsies in chronic rheumatic heart disease. 2. Muscle fiber reaction. *Pathol Res Pract* 179:600–609, 1985.

Virmani R, Roberts WC: Aschoff bodies in operatively excised atrial appendages and in papillary muscles: Frequency and clinical significance. *Circulation* 55:559–563, 1977.

Wagner BM, Tedeschi CG: Studies in rheumatic fever: II. Origin of cardiac giant cells. *Arch Pathol Lab Med* 60:423–430, 1955.

Wagner BM, Siew S: Studies in rheumatic fever. V. Significance of the human Anitschkow cell. *Hum Pathol* 1:45–71, 1970.

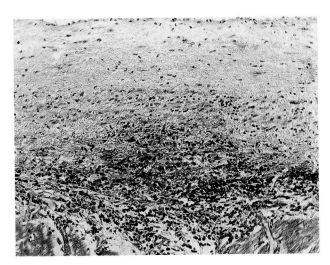

Figure 2.1. Early exudative type of an Aschoff body with central zone of fibrinoid necrosis.

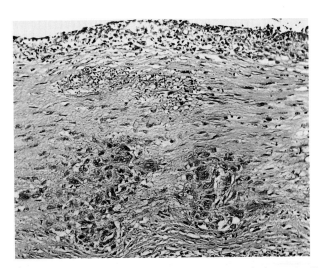

Figure 2.2. Two maturing subendocardial Aschoff bodies with clustering of myocardial histiocytes (Aschoff cells) and inflammatory exudate in the overlying endocardium.

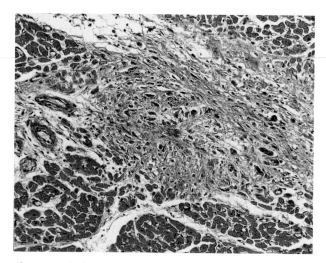

Figure 2.3. Typical perivascular location of an Aschoff body in rheumatic carditis.

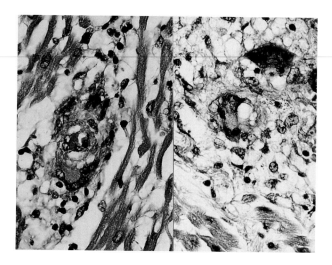

Figure 2.4. Aschoff giant cells in rheumatic carditis formed by coalesced myocardial histiocytes.

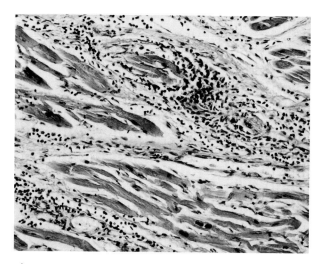

Figure 2.5. Nonspecific rheumatic myocarditis with lymphoplasmacytic infiltrate.

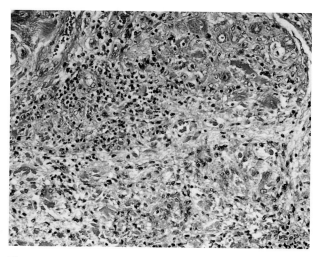

Figure 2.6. A granulomatous type of rheumatic myocarditis.

3. Rheumatoid Arthritis

Rheumatoid arthritis (RA) is a chronic, nonsuppurative, inflammatory polyarthritis of unknown cause affecting mainly the peripheral synovial joints, usually in a symmetrical fashion, with a prolonged course of exacerbation and remission, and often accompanied by symptoms and signs of a systemic disease.

Credit for the first description of what we now know as RA is often given to the French physician AJ Landré-Beauvais (1772–1840) who, in his Paris thesis of 1800, described nine women with a disease he considered a variant of gout and therefore called *goutte asthenique primitive.* It was Sir Alfred Garrod who first coined the term *rheumatoid arthritis* to distinguish it from gout; and Jean-Martin Charcot (1825–1893) also made clinical distinctions between gout, rheumatic fever, RA, and osteoarthritis, and first described pericarditis in 4 of 9 patients in 1881. The first roentgenogram of joints affected by RA was published by Gilbert A. Bannatyne in 1896 and, two years later, he reported involvement of peripheral nerves in RA with microscopic changes in the vasa nervorum—what might have been the first description of rheumatoid vasculitis. The modern concept of RA as a systemic disease was initiated in 1948 by Bauer and Clark's description of RA with extra-articular features and, in the same year, the term "rheumatoid disease" was coined by Ellman and Ball.

RA occurs worldwide. The most often cited prevalence rate is 1% in adult populations, but there is a wide variation of the reported rates from different ethnic groups and countries. The highest prevalence of RA has been found among some Native American populations and the lowest in certain Asian and African populations. The age distribution of RA is unimodal with peak age incidence between the fourth and sixth decades of life; women are two to three times more likely to develop RA than men. Compared with the age and gender matched control populations, mortality rates are increased at least two-fold in RA patients and the greater rates are linked to clinical severity of the disease and particularly among those whose disease began before 50 years of age. While the articular lesions of RA are disabling, the major cause of morbidity and mortality for those afflicted with the disease can be attributed largely to extra-articular manifestations of RA. Extra-articular manifestations tend to occur in patients who are seropositive, especially those with a higher rheumatoid factor titer and in whom the severity and duration of the disease are greater. With rare exceptions, biopsies in RA are directed to the diagnosis of extra-articular manifestations of the disease.

SYNOVIAL BIOPSY

Other than for research purposes and diagnosis of suspected coexisting joint disease, synovial biopsy is rarely carried out for confirmation of RA except when incidental to synovectomy as an elective surgical procedure. The key histologic features of rheumatoid synovitis comprise synoviocyte hyperplasia, subsynovial fibrosis, angiogenesis, perivascular lymphoplasmacytic infiltrate, and focal or diffuse aggregates of lymphocytes (Figs. 3.1 and 3.2). Among those patients with clinically active disease who have not received slow-acting disease-modifying drugs or intra-articular corticosteroids, there is considerable histopathologic homogeneity of the synovium within an individual diseased joint. However, in these patients no correlation could be found between the severity of any of the histopathologic features nor between any of these features and the extent of local joint damage, inflammation, or the severity of the systemic disease.

RHEUMATOID NODULES

Rheumatoid nodules are one of the best known characteristic features, but not a specific finding of RA. Necrobiotic nodules morphologically indistinguishable from the classic rheumatoid nodules occur in other rheumatic diseases as well as in patients without rheumatic symptoms or features, especially children, and in this latter group the lesions are known as benign rheumatoid nodulosis.

Rheumatoid nodules develop in about 20 to 30% of RA patients and are associated with circulating rheumatoid factors and with more severe erosive joint disease. The most common sites for rheumatoid nodules are the extensor surfaces of the arms and elbows, but they may be found anywhere in the subcutaneous tissue of the body, particularly on contact or pressure points over tendons and bones. They have also been described to occur, literally, from head to toes and all places in between: eye; bridge of the nose; pinna of the ear; larynx; pleura and lung; endocardium (including heart valves), myocardium, and pericardium; the abdominal wall and peritoneum; splenic capsule; over the ischial tuberosity and Achilles tendon.

A fully developed rheumatoid nodule comprises three zones: (a) a central area of necrosis often fibrinoid in appearance, surrounded by (b) a palisade of radially arranged elongated histiocytes which may have one or more nuclei, and (c) an outer layer of primarily a chronic granulation tissue with lymphocytes, plasma cells and proliferating fibroblasts. However, for a given rheumatoid nodule anywhere, the histologic feature of one or the other zones may predominate, and the mult-inucleated giant cells may be absent (Figs. 3.3 and 3.4).

Immunohistochemically, fibrin is abundant and small amounts of immunoglobulin can be identified in plasma cells and as extracellular deposits in and around the central zone of necrosis. Mononuclear cells around the zone of necrosis stain strongly positive with antisera to ferritin and a cytoplasmic macrophage antigen; stain variably with muramidase (lysozyme) and negatively with alpha-1-antitrypsin antibodies. Perls' stain for ferric iron is usually negative and ultrastructural x-ray micro-analysis indicates that the cytoplasm of these cells is also iron-free. These findings confirm the chronic in-flammatory nature of rheumatoid nodules but provide no support for the previously held view that they origi-nate in the vicinity of small vessel vasculitis.

Morris Ziff (1990) recently proposed that the process of rheumatoid nodule formation may consist of the fol-lowing possible steps: (1) trauma to small blood vessels with local pooling of rheumatoid factor immune com-plexes, (2) immune complex activation of local mono-cytes/macrophages causing the release of monocyte chemotactic factors, resulting in mobilization and recruitment of increased number of macrophages, (3) secretion of procoagulant by activated macrophages leading to fibrin deposition, (4) production of tissue necrosis by cytotoxic agents, proteinase, and collage-nases secreted by activated macrophages, and (5) assembly of palisading histiocytes around the central necrotic zone, mediated by macrophage-released chemotactic factor and interaction of the macrophage receptors with fibrin and fibronectin deposited at the margin of the zone of necrosis.

RHEUMATOID VASCULITIS

Up to 10% of RA patients may develop rheumatoid vas-culitis. Rheumatoid vasculitis occurs in blood vessels ranging in size from arterioles to the aorta (but most commonly in small and medium-sized arteries) and, thus, it produces a wide spectrum of clinical manifesta-tions. Clinical experience suggests that focal cutaneous lesions and isolated distal sensory neuropathy are not necessarily indicative of a poor prognosis, but multiple organ and visceral involvements are predictors of

increased morbidity and decreased actuarial survival of patients. Patients who develop rheumatoid vasculitis often have never taken disease-modifying drugs or have tolerated them poorly. This suggests the possibility that RA patients if treated early with disease-modifying drugs, including methotrexate, may be less and no more likely to develop rheumatoid vasculitis.

Rheumatoid vasculitis may occur in the early stage of the disease or, more frequently, in patients who have had seropositive RA for 10 years or longer. Homozy-gosity for the HLA-DRB1 0401 allele is common among patients with rheumatoid vasculitis. Clinical features and presentations of rheumatoid vasculitis include nail fold infarcts, leg ulcers, digital gangrene and peripheral neuropathy. With regard to peripheral neuropathy in rheumatoid vasculitis, a distal symmetric sensory or sensorimotor pattern occurs more commonly than mononeuritis multiplex. The inflammatory vascular dis-ease may be systemic, involving the visceromesenteric, coronary, and even cerebral arteries; these manifes-tations of rheumatoid vasculitis can occur singly or in variable combinations of different target vascular beds.

Although an assessment of the nature of vascular dis-ease in RA can sometimes be determined from clinical, laboratory, and angiographic examinations, biopsy con-firmation is necessary and recommended before sub-jecting the patient to immunosuppressive therapy. The biopsy site may be the symptomatic clinically involved tissue or other more accessible tissue; the latter includes the skeletal muscle, nerve, and rectum, probably in that order of preference, in RA patients suspected of having systemic vasculitis. In the absence of symptomatic sites, random or "blind" biopsies of the gastrocnemius muscle and/or the sural nerve are frequently practiced. Alterna-tively, the superficial branch of the peroneal nerve and the peroneus brevis muscle may be conveniently biop-sied on the same single procedure. In the vast majority of cases, light microscopic examination of multiple hematoxylin-eosin and elastin stain subserial or step sections (so as not to miss focal lesions) by a pathologist experienced in vasculitides would be all that is neces-sary. Immunohistochemical study of the muscle (for en-zymes or immune complexes) and ultrastructural study of the nerve (for axonal degeneration) are optional and become necessary only when indicated (Fig. 3.5).

Morphologically, a leukocytoclastic vasculitis typifies arteriolar and venular rheumatoid vasculitis (Fig. 3.6); the *acute* small and medium-sized arterial lesions, irre-spective of their location, are indistinguishable from the polyarteritis nodosa-type necrotizing vasculitis (Fig. 3.7) while the healed, *chronic* lesions are characterized by an endarteritis obliterans-type intimal fibrosis with scanty inflammatory cell infiltrate (Fig. 3.8). The large-vessel lesions are either a lymphoplasmacytic or granulomatous arteritis/aortitis (Figs. 3.9 and 3.10).

Muscle and/or nerve biopsies are currently the most common and useful procedures for histopathologic confirmation of rheumatoid vasculitis. According to a recently published French study (Puéchal et al. 1995), the following results of biopsy-documented rheumatoid vasculitis may be expected: arteritis is found only in the nerve biopsy in 14%; only in the muscle biopsy in 36%; and in both the nerve and muscle biopsies in 50%. Thus, for the combined procedure, the nerve biopsy is diagnostic in up to 64% and the muscle biopsy in up to 86% of RA patients with systemic rheumatoid vasculitis. Positive nerve biopsy for vasculitis can be expected with virtually the same frequency among patients with mainly sensory or mainly motor neuropathy; and positive nerve biopsy is not more frequent among those with the classic mononeuritis multiplex clinical presentation than in those with sensory or sensorimotor peripheral neuropathy.

RHEUMATOID HEART DISEASE

Nonspecific and specific cardiac lesions occur in RA. The reported clinical incidence of rheumatoid heart disease is highly variable, ranging from 3.4 to 34%; presumably in those series reporting low incidence the cardiac involvement may be overlooked in patients whose physical activity is restricted by RA and in whom chest discomfort may be masked by arthritic pains or modified by analgesics. The reported autopsy incidence is somewhat less variable: nonspecific pericarditis in 30–40%, myocarditis and valvular disease in 10–20%, and the specific rheumatoid nodules and rheumatoid vasculitis in any part of the heart in 5–20% of cases; it undoubtedly also indicates that cardiac lesions frequently persist whether or not the patients have clinically overt symptoms.

Acute (fibrinous) or chronic (fibrous) nonspecific pericarditis (Figs. 3.11 and 3.12) is the commonest form of cardiac involvement in RA; rheumatoid nodules are rarely found in the pericardium. The presence of pericarditis bears no relationship to the duration of RA, but it usually occurs in patients who have high-titer rheumatoid factor, subcutaneous nodules, and evidence of constitutional disease such as anemia and elevated erythrocyte sedimentation rate.

Two types of myocarditis may be found in RA patients with about equal frequency: one is a granulomatous myocarditis with or without necrobiotic rheumatoid nodules (Figs. 3.13 and 3.14), and the other is a nonspecific interstitial myocarditis with an infiltrate consisting of predominantly lymphocytes, plasma cells and histiocytes, and a variable number of eosinophils (Fig. 3.15). While most of the tissues removed at valve replacement surgery show fibrosis and calcification of end-stage disease, an occasional valve leaflet may still exhibit an apparent active valvulitis with necrobiotic rheumatoid nodules (Fig. 3.16). Coronary vasculitis in RA is seldom if ever a biopsy diagnosis, but it has been observed in 10–20% of autopsy patients.

RENAL AND HEPATIC DISORDERS

Glomerulonephritis is a rare complication of RA despite significant amounts of circulating immune complexes in both glomerulonephritis and RA. Nevertheless, renal failure is a frequent cause of death in RA patients, up to 20% in contrast with only 1% in the age and sex matched control population; most of the deaths are attributed to renal amyloidosis (Fig. 3.17).

There are no known hepatic diseases specific to RA. However, sequential liver biopsies are recommended for monitoring long-term methotrexate therapy-induced hepatotoxicity in RA patients. The important histopathologic findings in liver biopsies of graded severity include: anisonucleosis, bi- or trinucleations, focal necrosis, microvesicular steatosis, periportal bridging fibrosis, and portal hepatitis (Fig. 3.18).

RHEUMATOID LUNG DISEASE

Rheumatoid lung disease is probably the best known and most extensively studied pulmonary manifestation of rheumatic diseases, and it comprises a wide variety of clinicopathologic entities, all of which may be diagnosed in adequate (i.e., open) pleuropulmonary biopsies: (1) nonspecific or granulomatous pleuritis with or without effusion (Fig. 3.19); (2) necrobiotic rheumatoid nodules (Fig. 3.20); (3) rheumatoid pneumoconiosis (Caplan syndrome); (4) diffuse interstitial pneumonitis with fibrosis and sclerosing alveolitis (Fig. 3.21); (5) focal or diffuse lymphocytic interstitial pneumonitis (Fig.

3.22); (6) bronchiolitis obliterans and organizing pneumonitis; and (7) pulmonary vasculitis with or without pulmonary hypertension (Figs. 3.23 and 3.24). With the possible exceptions of the rheumatoid nodules and Caplan syndrome, none of the above-listed biopsy findings are specific for RA and the diagnosis of rheumatoid lung disease must be substantiated by or in accord with the appropriate clinical correlations.

BIBLIOGRAPHY

Aherne MJ, Bacon PA, Blake DR, et al: Immunohistochemical findings in rheumatoid nodules. *Virchows Arch Pathol Anat* 407:191–202, 1985.

Alarcón GS: Epidemiology of rheumatoid arthritis. *Rheum Dis Clin North Am* 21:589–604, 1995.

Anaya J-M, Diethelm L, Ortiz LA, et al: Pulmonary involvement in rheumatoid arthritis. *Semin Arthritis Rheum* 24:242–254, 1995.

Anthony DC, Crain BJ: Peripheral nerve biopsies. *Arch Pathol Lab Med* 120:26–34, 1996.

Bannatyne GA: *Rheumatoid Arthritis, Its Pathology, Morbid Anatomy, and Treatment,* ed 2. Bristol, John Wright, 1898, p 73.

Baggenstoss AH, Rosenberg EF: Cardiac lesions associated with chronic infectious (rheumatoid) arthritis. *Arch Intern Med* 67:241–248, 1941.

Baggenstoss AH, Rosenberg EF: Unusual cardiac lesions associated with chronic rheumatoid arthritis. *Arch Pathol* 37:54–60, 1944.

Ball J: Rheumatoid arthritis and polyarteritis nodosa. *Ann Rheum Dis* 13:277–290, 1954.

Bauer W, Clark WS: The systemic manifestations of rheumatoid arthritis. *Trans Assoc Am Physcns* 61:339–343, 1948.

Boers M: Renal disorders in rheumatoid arthritis. *Semin Arthritis Rheum* 20:57–68, 1990.

Bywaters EGL: Peripheral vascular obstruction in rheumatoid arthritis and its relationship to other vascular lesions. *Ann Rheum Dis* 16:84–103, 1957.

Cruickshank B: Heart lesions in rheumatoid disease. *J Pathol Bacteriol* 76:223–240, 1958.

Cathcart ES, Spodick DH: Rheumatoid heart disease: A study of the incidence and nature of cardiac lesions in rheumatoid arthritis. *N Engl J Med* 266:959–964, 1962.

Fingerman DL, Andrews FC: Visceral lesions associated with rheumatoid arthritis. *Ann Rheum Dis* 3:168–181, 1943.

Gardner DL: *Pathological Basis of the Connective Tissue Diseases.* Philadelphia, Lea & Febiger, 1992:444–526.

Geirsson AJ, Sturfelt G, Truedsson L: Clinical and serological features of severe vasculitis in rheumatoid arthritis: Prognostic implications. *Ann Rheum Dis* 46:727–733, 1987.

Gordon DA, Stein JL, Broder I: The extra-articular features of rheumatoid arthritis: A systemic analysis of 127 cases. *Am J Med* 54:445–452, 1973.

Gravallese EM, Corson JM, Coblyn JS, et al: Rheumatoid aortitis: A rarely recognized but clinically significant entity. *Medicine* 68:95–106, 1989.

Hakala M, Pääkko P, Huhti E, Tarkka M, Sutimen S: Open lung biopsy of patients with rheumatoid arthritis. *Clin Rheumatol* 9:452–460, 1990.

Hart FD: Rheumatoid arthritis: Extra-articular manifestations (Parts I and II). *Br Med J* 3:131–136, 1969; and 2:747–752, 1970.

Helin HJ, Korpela MM, Mustonen JT, Pasternack AI: Renal biopsy findings and clinico-pathologic correlations in rheumatoid arthritis. *Arthritis Rheum* 38:242–247, 1995.

Henderson DRF, Jayson MIV, Tribe CR: Lack of correlation of synovial histology with joint damage in rheumatoid arthritis. *Ann Rheum Dis* 34:7–11, 1977.

Hurd ER: Extraarticular manifestations of rheumatoid arthritis. *Semin Arthritis Rheum* 8:151–176, 1979.

Jordan JD: Cardiopulmonary manifestations of rheumatoid disease in childhood. *South Med J* 57:1273–1277, 1964.

Kay JM, Banik S: Unexplained pulmonary hypertension with pulmonary arteritis in rheumatoid disease. *Br J Dis Chest* 71:53–59, 1977.

Kaye BR, Kaye RL, Bobrove A: Rheumatoid nodules: Review of the spectrum of associated conditions and proposal of a new classification, with a report of four seronegative cases. *Am J Med* 76:279–292, 1984.

Kaye O, Beckers CC, Paquet P, et al: The frequency of cutaneous vasculitis is not increased in patients with rheumatoid arthritis treated with methotrexate. *J Rheumatol* 23:253–257, 1996.

Kremer JM, Kaye GI, Kaye KW, et al: Light and electron microscopic analysis of sequential liver biopsy samples from rheumatoid arthritis patients receiving long-term methotrexate therapy. *Arthritis Rheum* 38: 1194–1203, 1995.

Laakso M, Mutru O, Isomäki H, Koota K: Mortality from amyloidosis and renal diseases in patients with rheumatoid arthritis. *Ann Rheum Dis* 45:663–667, 1986.

Lakhanpal S, Conn DL, Lie JT: Clinical and prognostic significance of vasculitis as an early manifestation of connective tissue disease syndromes. *Ann Intern Med* 101:743–748, 1984.

Lie JT: Rheumatoid arthritis and heart disease. *Primary cardiol* 8(10):137–152, 1982.

Lie JT: Rheumatic connective tissue diseases. In Dail DH, Hammar SP (eds): *Pulmonary Pathology,* ed 2. New York, Springer-Verlag, 1994:679–705.

Lie JT: Pulmonary involvement in collagen vascular diseases. In Saldana M (ed): *Pathology of Pulmonary Disease.* Philadelphia, JB Lippincott Company, 1994: 781–790.

Myllykangas-Luosujärvi RA, Aho K, Isomäki HA: Mortality in rheumatoid arthritis. *Semin Arthritis Rheum* 25:193–202, 1995.

Padeh S, Laxer RM, Silver MM, Silverman ED: Primary pulmonary hypertension in a patient with systemic-onset juvenile arthritis. *Arthritis Rheum* 34:1575–1579, 1991.

Pagel W: Polyarteritis nodosa and the "rheumatic" diseases. *J Clin Pathol* 4:137–157, 1951.

Pincus T, Callahan LF: What is the natural history of rheumatoid arthritis? *Rheum Dis Clin North Am* 19: 123–151, 1993.

Puéchal X, Said G, Hilliquin P, et al: Peripheral neuropathy with necrotizing vasculitis in rheumatoid arthritis: A clinicopathologic and prognostic study of thirty-two patients. *Arthritis Rheum* 38:1618–1629, 1995.

Rooney M, Condell D, Quinlan W, et al: Analysis of the histologic variation of synovitis in rheumatoid arthritis. *Arthritis Rheum* 31:956–963, 1988.

Scott DGI, Bacon PA, Tribe CR: Systemic rheumatoid vasculitis: A clinical and laboratory study of 50 cases. *Medicine* 60:288–297, 1981.

Scott JT, Hourihane DO, Doyle FH, et al: Digital arteri-

tis in rheumatoid disease. *Ann Rheum Dis* 20: 224–234, 1961.

Sharma S, Vacharajani A, Mandke J: Severe pulmonary hypertension in rheumatoid arthritis. *Int J Cardiol* 26: 220–222, 1990.

Sokoloff L, Bunim JJ: Vascular lesions in rheumatoid arthritis. *J Chron Dis* 5:668–687, 1957.

Sokoloff L, McCluskey RT, Bunim JJ: Vascularity of the early subcutaneous nodule of rheumatoid arthritis. *Arch Pathol* 55:475–495, 1953.

Sokoloff L, Wilens SL, Bunim JJ: Arteritis of striated muscle in rheumatoid arthritis. *Am J Pathol* 27:157–173, 1951.

Stanley RJ, Subramanian R, Lie JT: Cholesterol pericarditis terminating as constrictive calcific pericarditis. *Am J Med* 45:511–514, 1980.

Symmons D: Excess mortality in rheumatoid arthritis—Is it the disease or the drug? *J Rheumatol* 22: 2200–2202, 1995.

Tribe CR: Amyloidosis in rheumatoid arthritis. *Modern Trend in Rheumatology.* London, Butterworths, 1966: 121.

Vollertsen RS, Conn DL: Vasculitis associated with rheumatoid arthritis. *Rheum Dis Clin North Am* 16: 445–461, 1990.

Vollertsen RS, Conn DL, Ballard DJ, et al: Rheumatoid vasculitis: Survival and associated risk factors. *Medicine* 65:365–375, 1986.

Voskuyl AE, Zwinderman AH, Westedt ML, et al: The mortality of rheumatoid vasculitis compared with rheumatoid arthritis. *Arthritis Rheum* 39:266–271, 1996.

Whaley K, Webb J: Liver and kidney disease in rheumatoid arthritis. *Clin Rheum Dis* 3:527–547, 1977.

Wolfe F, Mitchell DM, Sibley JT, et al: The mortality of rheumatoid arthritis. *Arthritis Rheum* 37:481–494, 1994.

Yousem SA, Colby TV, Carrington CB: Lung biopsy in rheumatoid arthritis. *Am Rev Respir Dis* 131: 770–777, 1985.

Ziff M: The rheumatoid nodule. *Arthritis Rheum* 33: 761–767, 1990.

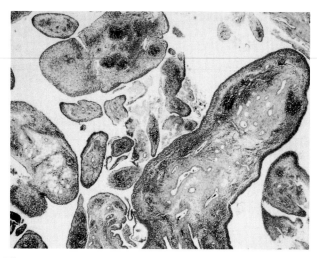

Figure 3.1. Villonodular synovitis with intense cellular infiltrates in rheumatoid arthritis.

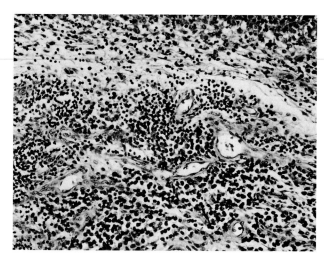

Figure 3.2. Higher magnification view of rheumatoid synovitis with angiogenesis and intense perivascular lymphoplasmacytic infiltrate.

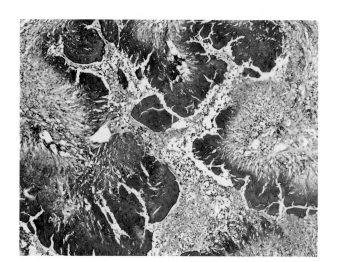

Figure 3.3. A rheumatoid nodule with fibrinoid central necrosis as a predominant feature.

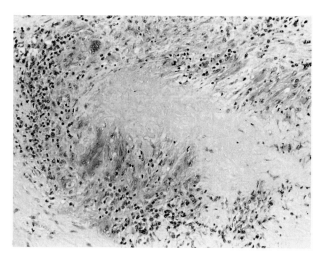

Figure 3.4. A typical rheumatoid nodule with peripheral palisading histiocytes and giant cells.

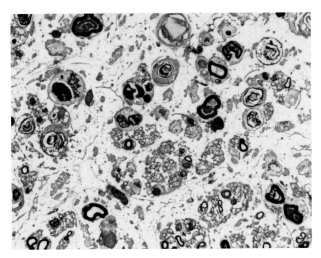

Figure 3.5. One-micron thick epon-embedded nerve biopsy specimen showing axonal degeneration of most fibers due to necrotizing vasculitis. *(Courtesy of Dr. Xavier Puéchal)*

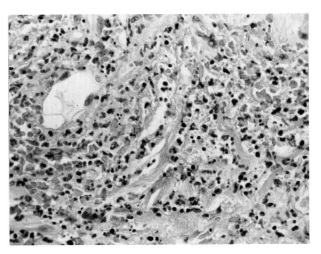

Figure 3.6. Cutaneous small-vessel leukocytoclastic vasculitis in rheumatoid arthritis.

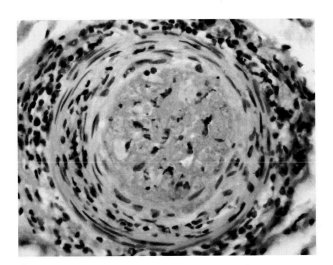

Figure 3.7. Small and medium-sized artery acute rheumatoid vasculitis is morphologically indistinguishable from polyarteritis nodosa-type necrotizing vasculitis.

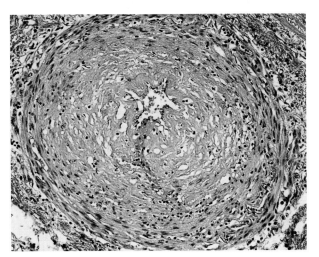

Figure 3.8. Chronic rheumatoid vasculitis resembling healed polyarteritis nodosa.

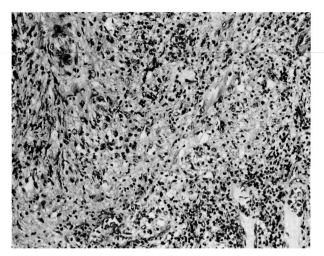

Figure 3.9. Inflammatory infiltrate of a lymphoplasmacytic aortitis in rheumatoid arthritis.

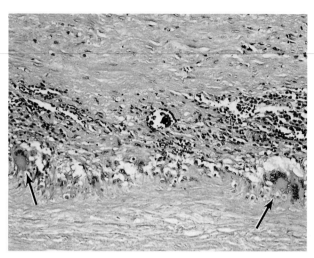

Figure 3.10. A granulomatous aortitis with giant cells *(arrows)* in rheumatoid arthritis.

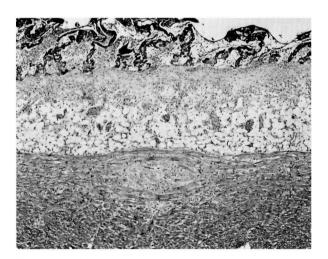

Figure 3.11. Nonspecific acute fibrinous pericarditis of rheumatoid arthritis.

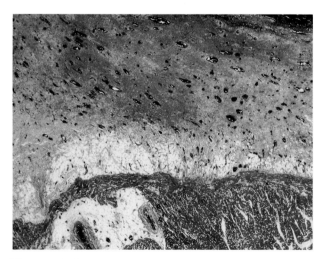

Figure 3.12. Nonspecific chronic fibrous pericarditis of rheumatoid arthritis with vascular granulation tissue in the thickened epicardium.

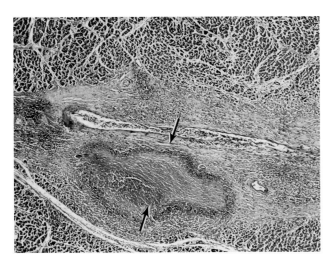

Figure 3.13. Granulomatous myocarditis in rheumatoid arthritis with an intramyocardial rheumatoid nodule *(arrows)*.

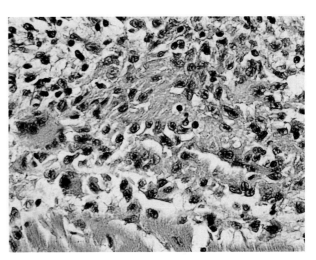

Figure 3.14. Granulomatous myocarditis in rheumatoid arthritis with an infiltrate consisting of lymphocytes, plasma cells, histiocytes, and giant cells.

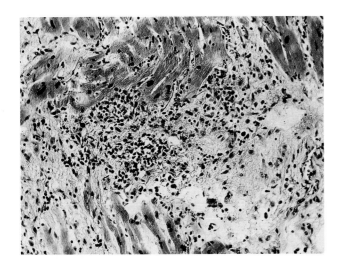

Figure 3.15. A nonspecific interstitial myocarditis in rheumatoid arthritis.

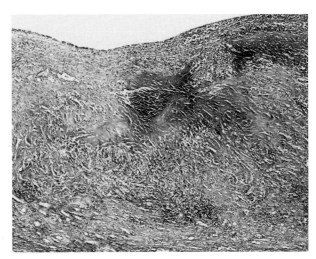

Figure 3.16. Excised mitral valve leaflet at valve replacement showing active granulomatous valvulitis with necrobiotic rheumatoid nodules.

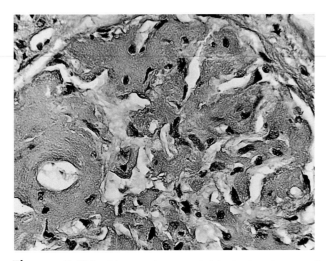

Figure 3.17. Glomerular amyloidosis in the renal biopsy of a rheumatoid arthritis patient.

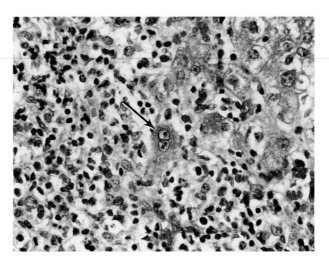

Figure 3.18. Liver biopsy of a rheumatoid arthritis patient on long-term methotrexate therapy, showing portal hepatitis with anisonucleosis and a binucleated hepatocyte *(arrow)*.

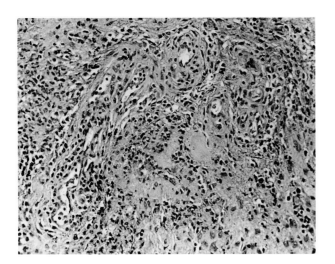

Figure 3.19. Granulomatous pleuritis without necrobiotic nodule in rheumatoid arthritis.

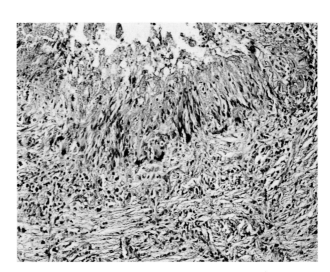

Figure 3.20. The edge of a pulmonary necrobiotic nodule in rheumatoid arthritis.

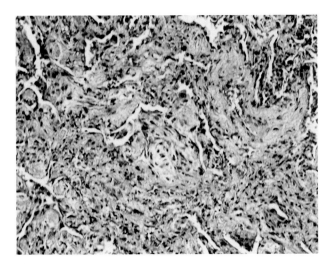

Figure 3.21. Diffuse interstitial pneumonitis with sclerosing alveolitis in rheumatoid arthritis.

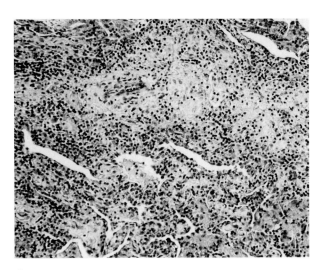

Figure 3.22. Diffuse lymphocytic interstitial pneumonitis in rheumatoid arthritis.

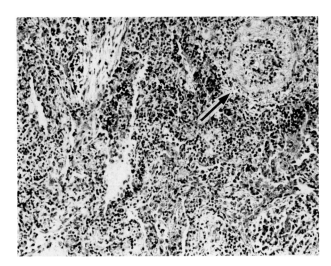

Figure 3.23. Lung biopsy with vasculitis *(arrow)* but without pulmonary hypertension in rheumatoid arthritis.

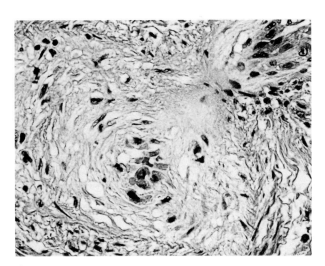

Figure 3.24. Lung biopsy with pulmonary hypertension (arterial pressure 76 mm Hg) vascular disease in rheumatoid arthritis.

4. Systemic Lupus Erythematosus

Lupus erythematosus was first described by the Austrian dermatologist Ferdinand von Hebra (1816–1880), in 1845, as *seborrhea congestiva,* a skin eruption that occurs " . . . mainly on the face, on the cheek and nose in a distribution not dissimilar to a butterfly." It was the French physician Pierre Louis Alphée Cazenave (1795–1877) who gave the disease its present name "lupus érythémateux" in 1851. Another Austrian dermatologist Moritz Kaposi-Kohn (1837–1902), in 1872, pointed out that the disease sometimes had systemic complications and was at times fatal. Many of the visceral manifestations of systemic lupus erythematosus (SLE) were described by William Osler (1849–1919) in a series of three articles published in 1895, 1900, and 1904. In 1924, Emanuel Libman and Benjamin Sacks at the Mount Sinai Hospital in New York added "atypical verrucous endocarditis" to the syndrome of SLE. From the same institution, Baehr, Klemperer, and Schifrin, in 1935, published a study of 23 autopsied cases (the largest series to that time) and described, in addition to the verrucous endocarditis, renal and extrarenal vascular disease and the "wire loop" glomerular lesions of SLE. Now, it has become all too familiar to us that virtually any and many organs may be involved in SLE (Table 4.1).

CUTANEOUS INVOLVEMENT

The lesions of discoid lupus erythematosus (DLE) are limited to the skin; serologic, hematologic and systemic abnormalities are slight or absent. Transition from a well established DLE to SLE with potentially serious or fatal outcome may occur but very rarely. Differentiation between DLE and SLE with a skin biopsy is generally not possible, because the skin lesions of DLE and SLE are not dissimilar and lesions having the typical histopathologic appearance of DLE can occur in SLE; a skin biopsy is therefore seldom carried out for the diagnosis of SLE. Furthermore, typical cutaneous lesions often are lacking early in the course of SLE, and in about 20% of the cases are absent throughout the course of the disease.

In most DLE lesions a diagnosis is possible based on a combination of histologic changes in the skin: (1) hyperkeratosis with keratotic plugging; (2) atrophy of the stratum malpighii; (3) hydropic degeneration of the basal cells; (4) a patchy and chiefly lymphoid cell infiltrate about the cutaneous appendages; and (5) edema, vasodilatation, and mild extravasation of erythrocytes in the upper dermis. Not all five changes are present in every case (Fig. 4.1).

In well developed cutaneous lesions of SLE, the histologic changes are similar to those of the erythematous and edematous lesions of DLE with additional findings of nonspecific perivascular fibrinoid deposits and lymphoid infiltrates in the dermis (Fig. 4.2). The fibrinoid deposits are PAS-positive and diastase-resistant, often found in areas exhibiting increased amounts of mucoid substance which stains positively with alcian blue and shows metachromasia on staining with toluidine blue. The subcutaneous fat may show mucoid degeneration with a reactive lymphocytic infiltrate, often referred to as *lupus panniculitis.*

CENTRAL NERVOUS SYSTEM INVOLVEMENT

Clinically, depending on the methods for detection and presence or absence of neurological symptoms, central nervous system (CNS) involvement occurs in 25–75% of reported series of SLE patients. The lack of reliable laboratory markers for CNS abnormalities and the limitation of ancillary procedures make the diagnosis of CNS involvement difficult. Moreover, differentiation between primary CNS lupus and CNS manifestations secondary to uremia, hypertension, CNS infection or drug treatment side effects is seldom conclusive.

Several studies have shown that brain magnetic resonance imaging (MRI) is a sensitive method of detecting anatomical abnormalities in periventricular or subcortical white matter and in grey matter, but up to 30–45% of CNS lupus patients may have normal scans. White matter lesions on MRI are not diagnostic of CNS lupus. Periventricular lesions are characteristic of multiple sclerosis, albeit more extensive and frequently in infratentorial locations; they have also been described in the acquired immune deficiency syndrome encephalopathy, Behçet's disease, sarcoidosis, Sjögren syndrome, Sneddon syndrome, and cerebral vasculitis.

Neuropathological studies in CNS lupus patients have seldom documented specific histologic findings. True cerebral vasculitis is rare, occurring probably in less than 5% of CNS lupus patients (Fig. 4.3), small-vessel perivascular and subcortical inflammatory infiltrates appear somewhat more common and have been loosely referred to as "cerebritis" (Fig. 4.4). Small infarcts with arteriolar and arterial occlusion, fibrinoid de-

Table 4.1. Frequency of Clinical Manifestations of Systemic Lupus Erythematosus*

Fever	90%
Weight loss	>80%
Skin lesions	>80%
Joint lesions	>80%
Renal disease	>50%
Neuropsychiatric disorders	>50%
Hematologic abnormalities	±50%
Cardiac involvement	±50%
Pulmonary involvement	±50%
Gastrointestinal involvement	±50%
Polyserositis	±10%

*Adapted with modification from Grishman et al (1993).

generation, hyalinization with necrosis and microglial proliferation occur less frequently. Changes in the CNS small blood vessels alone are not sufficient to account for most of the neuropsychiatric manifestations of CNS lupus.

Histopathologic studies of brains in elderly people with CNS lesions on MRI have shown dilated perivascular spaces and vascular ectasia, which are more often associated with arteriosclerosis, focal gliosis and demyelination, than with small cerebral infarcts. Punctate areas of increased signal on MRI in SLE probably represent edema, fluid-filled dilated perivascular spaces, gliosis, demyelination, mild nonspecific inflammatory changes and vasculopathy similar to that observed in elderly people. Cerebral atrophy is also a common MRI and computerized tomography (CT) finding in one-half to two-thirds of SLE patients, and it appears to be related to disease duration and long-term or high dose corticosteroid therapy. Vascular thromboembolic disease occurs more commonly in antiphospholipid syndrome associated with SLE (*vide infra*).

RENAL INVOLVEMENT

Renal disease is a major clinical problem accounting for significant morbidity and mortality in SLE patients. A renal biopsy finding of lupus nephritis is more frequent than abnormal urinalysis or abnormal creatinine clearance. Renal involvement occurs more commonly in SLE patients under 30 years of age and develops earlier in the course of the disease in these patients; and it may

include the entire spectrum of glomerular, tubular, or vascular diseases. The onset may be quite insidious or precipitous with nephrotic syndrome as the most common presentation, and the course may be brief, but more often it progresses to chronic renal failure. In general, the severity of morphologic lesions parallels that of clinical renal disease, and the course of lupus nephritis is influenced by the severity of the underlying lesions and the type of therapy given.

Classifications have been devised to gauge the severity of glomerular histopathologic changes and correlate them with the clinical outcome. The most widely used World Health Organization (WHO) classification divides lupus nephritis into six classes (Table 4.2), and a scoring system has also been developed to provide indices of activity and chronicity in individual cases (Table 4.3). Lupus nephritis is a specialized topic of renal pathology, the readers are referred to two recently published monographs, one by Grishman et al. (1993) and one by Churg et al. (1995) for detailed description and an Atlas of glomerular diseases in SLE, respectively.

Table 4.2. Modified WHO Classification of Lupus Nephritis in Renal Biopsies*

Class I	Normal glomeruli (by all techniques)
Class II	Pure mesangial alterations (mesangiopathy)
	A: Immune deposits by immunofluorescence or electron microscopy
	B: Mesangial widening and variable hypercellularity
Class III	Focal segmental glomerulonephritis associated with mild or moderate mesangial alterations
	A: Active necrotizing lesions
	B: Active necrotizing and sclerosing lesions
	C: Sclerosing lesions
Class IV	Diffuse glomerulonephritis (severe mesangial, endocapillary, mesangiocapillary proliferation and/or subendothelial deposits)
	A: Without segmental lesions
	B: With active necrotizing lesions
	C: With active and sclerosing lesions
	D: With sclerosing lesions
Class V	Diffuse membranous glomerulonephritis
	A: Pure membranous glomerulonephritis
	B: Associated with lesions of Class II (A or B)
Class VI	Advanced sclerosing glomerulonephritis (end-stage disease)

*Adapted with modification from Grishman et al (1993) and Churg et al (1995).

Table 4.3. Activity and Chronicity indices of Lupus Nephritis*

Active Lesions
  A. Glomerular
     1. Cellular proliferation
     2. Disruption of capillary walls
     3. Polymorphs and karyorrhexis
     4. Hematoxyphil bodies
     5. Crescents, cellular or fibrocellular
     6. "Wire loops" (by light microscopy)
     7. Hyaline thrombi
     8. Fibrin thrombi
     9. Segmental fibrin deposition
  B. Vascular
     1. Hyaline (immune complex) deposits
     2. Necrotizing vasculitis
  C. Tubular degeneration and necrosis
  D. Interstitial inflammation, active
Sclerosing Lesions
  A. Glomerular sclerosis
     1. Segmental
     2. Mesangial
     3. Global
  B. Fibrous crescents
  C. Tubular atrophy
  D. Interstitial fibrosis
  E. Vascular sclerosis

*Modified from Grishman et al (1993) and Churg et al (1995).

There are two common types of renal vascular lesions in SLE: one is necrotizing arteritis and arteriolitis (Fig. 4.5) occurring usually in patients who have severe hypertension and progressive renal failure, and the other is "lupus vasculopathy" characterized by subendocardial deposition of eosinophilic PAS-positive proteinaceous material (Fig. 4.6) and consisting of an admixture of immunoglobulins and complement components, detectable by immunofluorescent microscopy. Occasionally, a thrombotic microangiopathy may be observed in renal biopsies.

CARDIOVASCULAR INVOLVEMENT

Moritz Kaposi-Kohn, who first considered SLE a systemic disease in 1872, provided the earliest known evidence of cardiovascular involvement in SLE when he mentioned cardiac irregularity in one patient and dyspnea in another. Libman and Sacks clearly distinguished the "atypical verrucous endocarditis" they described in 1924 from rheumatic and bacterial endocardial disease. They did not recognize the full significance of these lesions although they had also found cutaneous changes of lupus erythematosus in two of their four patients with the endocarditis. It was Louis Gross, also from New York's Mount Sinai Hospital, who first linked the Libman-Sacks endocarditis to SLE.

In almost one half of all SLE patients, cardiac involvement develops at some time during their illness but it may be asymptomatic clinically. Nonspecific pericarditis, nonbacterial verrucous endocarditis, and myocarditis occur in about 45%, 35%, and 25% of SLE patients, respectively. Pericarditis and endocarditis are seldom biopsied, but endomyocardial biopsy has been used increasingly frequently for the diagnosis of lupus myocarditis. Myocardial infarction or myocardial necrosis occurs in 10–15% of SLE patients under 50 years of age; the former lesion is caused by premature atherosclerosis or coronary thrombosis and the latter by immune complex mediated coronary vasculitis or microvascular thrombosis; and the thrombosis in both situations is often associated with the antiphospholipid syndrome.

Because of the sampling problem for focal lesions and the limited tissue fragment size, endomyocardial biopsies must be interpreted cautiously and with clinical correlation. The intensity of cell infiltrate in lupus myocarditis may be highly variable and cannot be equated with either the extent of involvement or the severity of disease (Figs. 4.7 and 4.8); and a negative biopsy with insufficient tissue fragments cannot rule out myocarditis. The cell infiltrate in lupus myocarditis is predominantly lymphocytic, to be distinguished from a healing infarct with a similar type of inflammatory infiltrate (Figs. 4.9 and 4.10).

The small-vessel inflammatory disease in SLE, irrespective of the vascular bed involved, is typically a polyarteritis-type necrotizing vasculitis (Figs. 4.3, 4.5, and 4.11). Large-vessel inflammatory disease, such as a lymphoplasmacytic or granulomatous aortitis (Fig. 4.12), occurs rarely in SLE and morphologically may be indistinguishable from Takayasu aortitis.

PULMONARY INVOLVEMENT

Although William Osler in 1904 had mentioned pulmonary consolidation and hemoptysis in a 24-year-old woman with SLE, specific pulmonary manifestations of SLE were first described by Rakov and Taylor in 1942.

The prevalence of pulmonary involvement in SLE varies widely according to subsequent reports, from 9% to 90%, and is probably more realistically in the 20–40% range; many of the pulmonary lesions previously attributed to SLE either could be explained by alternative causes or were unconfirmed histopathologically, and the latter depended on whether the tissue was obtained by transbronchial or open lung biopsy.

What might be the most specific lung biopsy finding in SLE, endovascular hematoxyphil bodies (Fig. 4.13), is also the rarest and obtainable only serendipitously. The nonspecific so-called "usual interstitial pneumonia" occurs in less than 10% of SLE patients; and when diffuse pulmonary fibrosis is found, one should question whether another connective tissue disease or an overlap syndrome might be the correct diagnosis. The possibility of pulmonary complications of antirheumatic drug therapy must also be considered in the differential diagnoses. Among the more recently described and still relatively uncommon pulmonary manifestations of SLE include bronchiolitis obliterans-organizing pneumonia (Fig. 4.14) and lymphocytic interstitial pneumonitis with or without pseudolymphoma (Fig. 4.15).

Vascular disease is, on the other hand, a much more common and important pulmonary manifestation of SLE. Diffuse alveolar hemorrhage (which at times may be fatal) secondary to pulmonary capillaritis (Fig. 4.16), pulmonary vasculitis (Fig. 4.17), which may be isolated or associated with plexogenic pulmonary hypertension (Fig. 4.18) are a major cause of morbidity and mortality in SLE. Immune complex deposits of IgG, IgM, IgA, and C3 have been demonstrated in the alveolar interstitium and blood vessel walls of the affected lungs.

BIBLIOGRAPHY

Abu-Shakra M, Gladman DD, Urowitz MB, Farewell V: Anticardiolipin antibodies in systemic lupus erythematosus: Clinical and laboratory correlations. *Am J Med* 99:624–628, 1995.

Abud-Mendoza C, Diaz-Jouanen E, Alarcón-Segovia D: Fatal pulmonary hemorrhage in systemic lupus erythematosus: Occurrence without hemoptysis. *J Rheumatol* 12:558–561, 1985.

Ansari A, Larson PH, Bates HD: Cardiovascular manifestations of systemic lupus erythematosus: Current perspective. *Progr Cardiovasc Dis* 27:421–434, 1985.

Ansari A, Larson PH, Bates HD: Vascular manifestations of systemic lupus erythematosus. *Angiology* 37: 423–432, 1986.

Asherson RA, Hackett D, Gharavi AE, et al: Pulmonary hypertension in systemic lupus erythematosus. *J Rheumatol* 13:416–420, 1986.

Baehr G, Klemperer P, Schifrin A: A diffuse disease of the peripheral circulation usually associated with lupus erythematosus and endocarditis. *Trans Assoc Am Physicians* 50:139–155, 1935.

Belmont HM, Abramson SB, Lie JT: Pathology and pathogenesis of vascular injury in systemic lupus erythematosus: Interactions of inflammatory cells and activated endothelium. *Arthritis Rheum* 39:9–22, 1996.

Bidani AK, Roberts JL, Schwartz MM, Lewis EJ: Immunopathology of cardiac lesions in fatal systemic lupus erythematosus. *Am J Med* 69:849–858, 1980.

Bluestone HG: Neuropsychiatric manifestations of systemic lupus erythematosus. *N Engl J Med* 317: 309–311, 1987.

Cervera R, Asherson RA, Lie JT: Clinicopathologic correlations of the antiphopholipid syndrome. *Semin Arthritis Rheum* 24:262–272, 1995.

Churg J, Bernstein J, Glassock RJ: *Renal Disease: Classification and Atlas of Glomerular Disease,* ed 2. New York, Igaku-Shoin, 1995:151–179.

Doherty NE, Siegel RJ: Cardiovascular manifestations of systemic lupus erythematosus. *Am Heart J* 110: 1257–1265, 1985.

Esdaile JM, Joseph L, MacKenzie T, et al: The pathogenesis and prognosis of lupus nephritis: Information from repeat renal biopsy. *Semin Arthritis Rheum* 23: 135–148, 1993.

Ellis SG, Verity MA: Central nervous system involvement in systemic lupus erythematosus: A review of neuropathological findings in 57 cases, 1955–1977. *Semin Arthritis Rheum* 8:212–221, 1979.

Fearon WF, Cooke JP: Acute myocardial infarction in a young woman with systemic lupus erythematosus. *Vasc Med* 1:19–23, 1996.

Galve E, Candell-Riera J, Pigrau C, et al: Prevalence, morphologic types, and evolution of cardiac valvular disease in systemic lupus erythematosus. *N Engl J Med* 319:817–823, 1988.

Gardner DG: *Pathological Basis of the Connective Tissue Diseases.* Philadelphia, Lea & Febiger, 1992: 568–613.

Gilliam JN, Sontheimer RD: Skin manifestations of SLE. *Clin Rheum Dis* 8:207–218, 1981.

Gonzalez-Crespo MR, Blanco FJ, Ramos A, et al: Magnetic resonance imaging of the brain in systemic lupus erythematosus. *Br J Rheumatol* 34:1055–1060, 1995.

Grishman E, Churg J, Needle MA, Venkataseshan VS (eds): *The Kidney in Collagen-Vascular Diseases.* New York, Raven Press 1993:45–86.

Gross L: The cardiac lesions in Libman-Sacks disease: With a consideration of its relationship to acute diffuse lupus erythematosus. *Am J Pathol* 16:375–407, 1940.

Haupt HM, Moore GW, Hutchins GM: The lung in systemic lupus erythematosus: Analysis of the pathologic changes in 120 patients. *Am J Med* 71:791–798, 1981.

Hejtmancik MR, Wright JC, Quint R, Jennings FL: The cardiovascular manifestations of systemic lupus erythematosus. *Am Heart J* 68:119–130, 1954.

Homcy CJ, Liberthson RR, Fallon JJ, et al: Ischemic heart disease in systemic lupus erythematosus in the young patient. *Am J Med* 49:478–484, 1982.

Kaposi-Kohn M: Neue Beiträge zur Kenntnis des Lupus erythematosus. *Arch Dermatol Syphil* (Prague) 4: 36–78, 1872.

Leatherman JW: Immune alveolar hemorrhage. *Chest* 91:891–897, 1987.

Lewis EJ, Kawala K, Schwartz MM: Histologic features that correlate with the progression of patients with lupus nephritis. *Am J Kidney Dis* 10:192–197, 1987.

Libman E, Sacks B: A hitherto undescribed form of vascular and mural endocarditis. *Arch Intern Med* 33: 701–737, 1924.

Lie JT: Systemic and isolated vasculitis: A rational approach to classification and pathologic diagnosis. *Pathol Annu* 24 (part 1):25–114, 1989.

Lie JT: Rheumatic connective tissue diseases. In Dail DH, Hammar SP (eds): *Pulmonary Pathology,* ed 2. New York, Springer-Verlag, 1994:679–705.

Lie JT: Pulmonary involvement in collagen vascular diseases. In Saldana M (ed): *Pathology of Pulmonary Disease.* Philadelphia, JB Lippincott Company, 1994: 781–790.

Lie JT, Kobayashi S, Tokano Y, Hashimoto H: Systemic and cerebral vasculitis coexisting with disseminated coagulopathy in systemic lupus erythematosus associated with antiphospholipid syndrome. *J Rheumatol* 22:2173–2176, 1995.

Lie JT: Pathology of the antiphospholipid syndrome. In Asherson RA, Cervera R, Piette JC, Schoenfeld Y (eds): *The Antiphospholipid Syndrome.* Boca Raton, FL, CRC Press, 1996:89–104.

Mandell BF: Cardiovascular involvement in systemic lupus erythematosus. *Semin Arthritis Rheum* 17: 126–141, 1987.

Miller DH, Ormerod LEC, Gibson A, et al: MRI brain scanning in patients with vasculitis: Differentiation from multiple sclerosis. *Neuroradiology* 29:226–231, 1987.

Myers JL, Katzenstein AL: Microangiitis in lupus-induced pulmonary hemorrhage. *Am J Clin Pathol* 85:552–556, 1986.

Nossent HC, Henzen-Logmans SC, Vroom TM, et al: Contribution of renal biopsy data in predicting outcome in lupus nephritis. *Arthritis Rheum* 33: 970–977, 1990.

Orens JB, Martinez FJ, Lynch JP III: Pleuropulmonary manifestations of systemic lupus erythematosus. *Rheum Dis Clin North Am* 20:159–193, 1994.

Osler W: On the visceral complications of erythema exudativum multiforme. *Am J Med Sci* 110:629–646, 1895.

Osler W: On the visceral manifestations of erythema group of skin diseases. *Am J Med Sci* 127:1–23, 1904.

Petri M, Perez-Gutthann S, Spence D, Hochberg MC: Risk factors for coronary artery disease in patients with systemic lupus erythematosus. *Am J Med* 93: 513–519, 1992.

Rakov HL, Taylor JS: Acute disseminated lupus erythematosus without cutaneous manifestations and heretofore undescribed pulmonary lesions. *Arch Intern Med* 70:88–100, 1942.

Schwab EP, Schumacher HR, Freundlich B, Calligari PE: Pulmonary alveolar hemorrhage in systemic lupus erythematosus. *Semin Arthritis Rheum* 23:8–15, 1993.

Segal AM, Calabrese L, Ahmad M, et al: The pulmonary manifestations of systemic lupus erythematosus. *Semin Arthritis Rheum* 14:202–224, 1985.

Straaton KV, Chatham WW, Reveille JD, et al: Clinically significant valvular heart disease in systemic lupus erythematosus. *Am J Med* 85:645–650, 1988.

Sturfelt G, Eskilsson J, Nived O, Truedsson L, Valina S: Cardiovascular disease in systemic lupus erythematosus. *Medicine* 71:216–223, 1992.

Tsumagari T, Fukumoto S, Mitsuru K, Kenzo T: Incidence and significance of intrarenal vasculopathies in patients with systemic lupus erythematosus. *Hum Pathol* 16:43–49, 1989.

Ward MM, Pyun E, Studenski S: Cause of death in systemic lupus erythematosus: Long-term followup of an inception cohort. *Arthritis Rheum* 38:1492–1499, 1995.

Wilson VE, Eck SL, Bates EB: Evaluation and treatment of acute myocardial infarction complicating systemic lupus erythematosus. *Chest* 101:420–424.

Yoshio T, Masuyama J, Sumiya M, et al: Antiendothelial cell antibodies and their relation to pulmonary hypertension in systemic lupus erythematosus. *J Rheumatol* 21: 2058–2063, 1994.

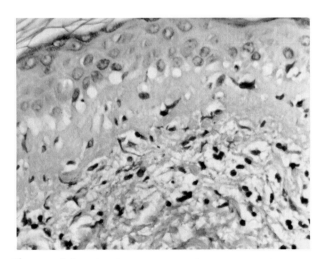

Figure 4.1. Skin biopsy in SLE showing atrophy of the stratum malpighii and hydropic degeneration of the basal cells.

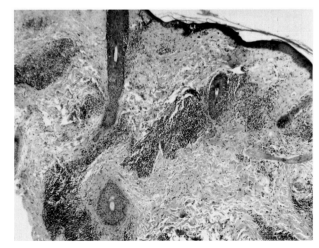

Figure 4.2. Skin biopsy in SLE showing interstitial fibrinoid deposits and perivascular lymphocytic infiltrate.

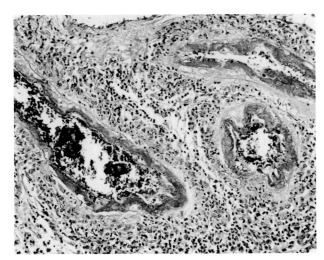

Figure 4.3. Brain biopsy in CNS lupus showing necrotizing vasculitis in meninges.

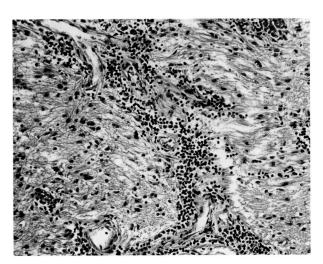

Figure 4.4. Brain biopsy in CNS lupus showing perivascular and subcortical lymphocytic infiltrate without true vasculitis ("cerebritis").

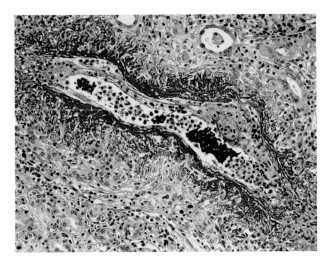

Figure 4.5. Polyarteritis-type necrotizing vasculitis in SLE renal biopsy.

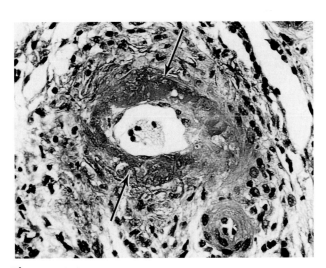

Figure 4.6. Renal microvascular angiopathy in SLE with subendothelial PAS-positive amorphous protein deposits (*arrows*).

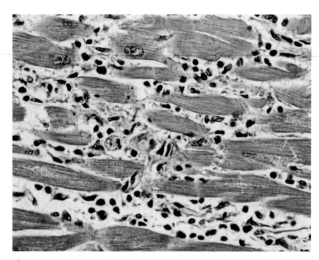

Figure 4.7. Lupus myocarditis with mild to moderate inflammatory infiltrate.

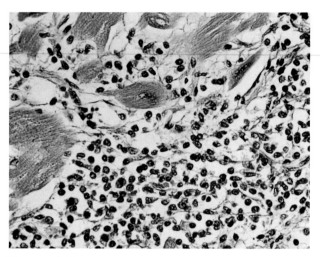

Figure 4.8. Lupus myocarditis with more intense lymphoplasmacytic infiltrate.

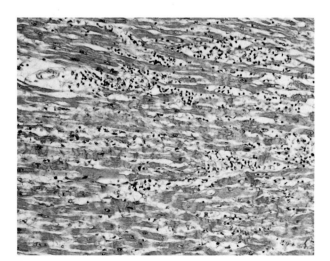

Figure 4.9. Lupus myocarditis with endomyocardial biopsy-related contraction bands artefact but without fibrosis of a healing infarct.

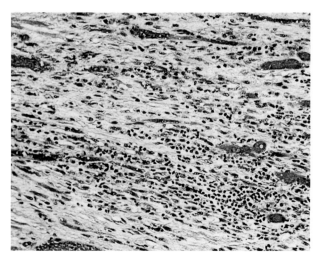

Figure 4.10. Biopsy finding of a healing infarct with fibrosis and an inflammatory infiltrate.

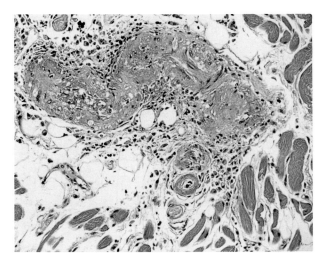

Figure 4.11. Intramyocardial polyarteritis-type small vessel necrotizing vasculitis in SLE.

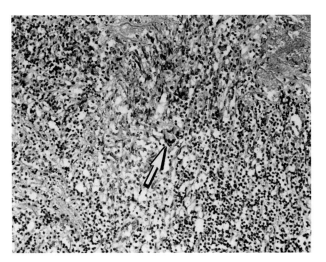

Figure 4.12. Granulomatous aortitis with giant cells (*arrow*) in SLE indistinguishable from Takayasu aortitis. (Biopsy obtained at repair of ascending aortic aneurysm with dissection)

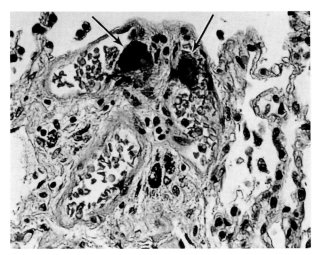

Figure 4.13. Pulmonary endovascular hematoxyphil bodies (*arrows*) in biopsy of lupus lung.

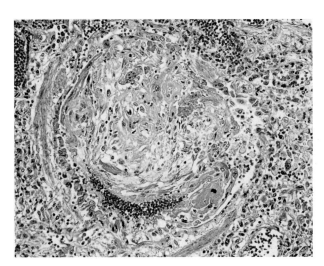

Figure 4.14. Bronchiolitis obliterans in biopsy of lupus lung.

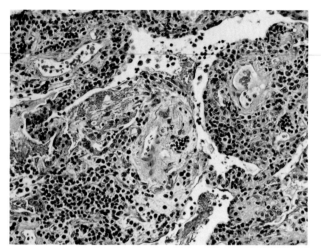

Figure 4.15. Lymphocytic interstitial pneumonitis in biopsy of lupus lung.

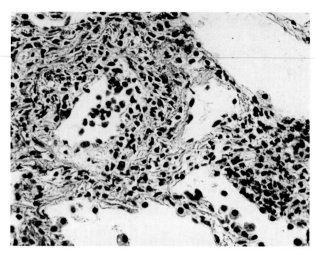

Figure 4.16. Pulmonary capillaritis in biopsy of lupus lung.

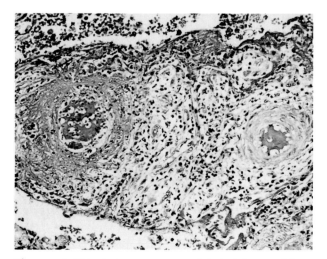

Figure 4.17. Pulmonary vasculitis in biopsy of lupus lung.

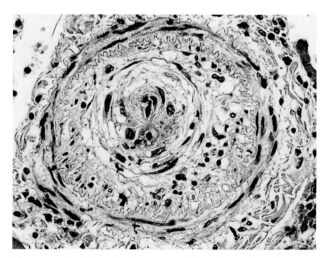

Figure 4.18. Plexiform arteriopathy of pulmonary hypertension in lupus lung.

5. Scleroderma and the CREST Syndrome

Scleroderma, a clinical term suggested by the French physician Elie Gintrac (1791–1877) in 1847, was first used to describe a disease characterized by hard tight skin with a hidebound appearance. Later, it became apparent that scleroderma could have systemic involvement manifested by diffuse connective tissue and/or vascular alterations. Maurice Raynaud (1834–1881) first described the vasospastic phenomenon that bears his name in 1862 and, in 1863, he commented on its occurrence in a patient with scleroderma. In the same year, Heinrich Auspitz (1835–1886) described the case of a locksmith with sclerodactyly who died of acute renal failure, but renal involvement was considered a chance association with scleroderma until 1952 when Moore and Sheehan provided the first detailed report of renal complications of scleroderma. Subsequently, in 1957, Rodnan et al. reported nine scleroderma patients with renal involvement, seven of whom died in acute renal failure.

Based on the distribution and extent of skin involvement and the presence of visceral involvement, a distinction can be made between *limited* and *diffuse* (or systemic) forms of scleroderma. The systemic form has been referred to in the past as *progressive systemic sclerosis* (PSS); however, this term was recently discarded in favor of *systemic sclerosis* (SSc) because not all cases are progressive but most remain clinically stable for many years. Other connective tissue diseases (such as rheumatoid arthritis, systemic lupus erythematosus, dermatomyositis, and Sjögren's syndrome) may sometimes be associated with SSc, and these conditions are referred to as *overlap syndromes.*

Patients with the limited form of SSc tend to be older and typically have a longer history of Raynaud phenomenon, often associated with facial telangiectasias and skin thickening of distal extremities. Over the course of many years, esophageal hypomotility and interstitial lung disease may ensue, but renal involvement seldom occurs. This variant of SSc is known as the CREST syndrome; the acronym stands for *c*alcinosis, *R*aynaud phenomenon, *e*sophageal dysfunction, *s*clerodactyly, and *t*elangiectasias. Patients with the CREST syndrome may be distinguished serologically from those with SSc by their high (70–80%) incidence of anticentromere antibody and absence of antitopoisomerase antibody.

Scleroderma occurs worldwide, and is primarily a disease of middle- and late middle-aged women. The overall female/male incidence ratio is 3:1 but it rises to 15:1 during the childbearing age of 20–45 years. Scleroderma is rare in children, with perhaps fewer than 100 cases reported in the literature up to 1990. The standardized mortality ratios (SMR) calculated for 237 patients with SSc followed prospectively for 15 years (1976–1990) in a Canadian study was 4.69. The mortality rate was greater with diffuse than limited SSc (SMR 6.18 and 3.80, respectively), but not different between men and women. Renal, cardiac, pulmonary, and gastrointestinal involvement predicted reduced survival in diffuse SSc, when compared with the general population.

SKIN, DIGESTIVE TRACT, AND MUSCLE INVOLVEMENT

Scleroderma and the CREST syndrome owe their names to the early clinical recognition and easy detection of cutaneous, gastrointestinal, and muscular manifestations in these disorders. However, a skin biopsy is seldom necessary for the diagnosis of the disease, and pathologic examination of the esophagus or intestinal tract is performed only on tissue samples obtained incidental to surgical interventions for complications of SSc.

A typical SSc skin biopsy is characterized by thinning of the epidermis with loss of rete pegs, marked increase of compact collagen fibers in the dermis with vanishing dermal adnexal structures, and vessel wall hyalinization and luminal obliteration of arterioles (Fig. 5.1). Telangiectasia, consisting of dilated capillaries and subpapillary venule plexus, may develop on the facial skin, oral mucosa, nailfolds and fingers. Histologic examination of digital arteries in SSc patients with Raynaud's phenomenon and peripheral ischemia typically shows a bland occlusive intimal fibrocellular proliferation with or without a concomitant organized thrombus (Fig. 5.2).

Direct gross examination and motility study of the esophagus may reveal atrophy of the muscularis and tubular shortening from the mid-segment to the cardia; the upper portion of the esophagus escapes most of the regressive changes. Ulcers and diverticula are known to occur in the esophagus, stomach, small bowel and colon, presumably resulting from edema, intimal fibrosis and degenerative changes of the blood vessels in the wall of the hollow viscus. The myenteric plexus in the esophagus and colon may be deficient or lacking in ganglion cells. Atrophy of the muscularis mucosa may allow air or gas entry into the bowel wall and the development of pneumatosis cystoides intestinalis (Fig. 5.3).

Skeletal muscle involvement in SSc is uncommon and shows considerable variability. Muscle biopsy is performed infrequently, and usually more for the exclusion of other disease than for the diagnosis of SSc. The changes observed range from no abnormality to myositis with predominantly a lymphocytic infiltrate to myocyte atrophy and interstitial fibrosis. The myositis is usually seen in SSc patients with symptoms and clinical findings that overlap those of dermatomyositis, the so-called "sclerodermatomyositis." Expression of neural cell adhesion molecule in atrophic fibers can be demonstrated histochemically in muscle biopsies of patients with progressive muscle weakness (Fig. 5.4).

RENAL INVOLVEMENT

The incidence of renal disease in SSc is difficult to determine because of biases in patient referral pattern, diagnostic criteria, and the preponderance of autopsy-based studies favoring selection of patients with end-stage disease; the best estimate is in the range of 30–60%.

The renal biopsy findings in SSc patients range from minimal involvement to severe and life-threatening changes. A distinctive feature of scleroderma kidney is occlusive vascular disease of arterioles and interlobular small arteries with an external diameter of 150–500 μm by edematous mucoid intimal proliferation, sometimes with fibrinoid necrosis of the vessel wall, which is morphologically indistinguishable from the small vessel changes of malignant hypertension (Fig. 5.5). Rarely, larger-caliber arteries show occlusive, concentric onion-skin pattern intimal myointimal cell proliferation. The acute glomerular disease is characterized by capillary occlusion with fibrin thrombi (Fig. 5.6), and ischemic changes signify chronic disease; neither is specific for scleroderma but the diagnosis is aided by the concomitant telltale arterial and arteriolar vasculopathy.

CARDIOVASCULAR MANIFESTATIONS

There are no specific cardiac lesions of scleroderma, as observed in endomyocardial biopsies. A common finding is sclerosing occlusive small vessel disease of intramural branches of the coronary arteries, often associated with prominent interstitial fibrosis and dilated lymphatics (Fig. 5.7). Similar changes have been observed in the cardiac conduction tissue of autopsied hearts and invoked as a possible cause of heart block in SSc patients. A less common biopsy finding is myocarditis which, according to some investigators, often occurs in SSc patients who have an inflammatory skeletal myopathy indistinguishable from that of polymyositis. An unconfirmed observation of myocarditis in SSc is the frequent occurrence of "contraction band necrosis" or "myofibrillar degeneration" (Fig. 5.8).

Vasculitis has seldom been reported as a complication of scleroderma. In the classic case-control autopsy study of D'Angelo et al., 5 of 58 SSc patients had acute necrotizing vasculitis morphologically similar to polyarteritis nodosa involving vessels in several organ systems. One of these patients had systemic lupus erythematosus and another had classic rheumatoid arthritis. Even more uncommon are reports of large vessel occlusive disease involving principally the brachiocephalic and ilio-femoro-popliteal arteries. The cause is unknown, possibly because most of these cases were diagnosed clinically or angiographically without histopathologic confirmation.

SCLERODERMA LUNG DISEASE

As is with renal involvement, SSc patients with pulmonary involvement have significantly poorer survival prospects. Histologic evaluation of scleroderma lung disease until recently had been based on the results of autopsy studies which emphasized the end-stage fibrosis associated with bronchiectasis and subpleural honey-combing (Fig. 5.9). The earlier phase of interstitial lung disease in scleroderma, as seen in open biopsies, is indistinguishable from the idiopathic usual interstitial pneumonitis, or UIP (Fig. 5.10). However, interstitial fibrosis in scleroderma tends to be indolent and more slowly progressive than UIP. A more rapidly progressive diffuse alveolar damage and bronchiolitis obliterans (Fig. 5.11) is a less common manifestation of scleroderma lung disease.

Proliferative arteriopathy is a common and important manifestation of scleroderma lung disease, which may or may not be associated with pulmonary hypertension. Pulmonary hypertension occurs in an estimated 10–35% of SSc patients and in 40–65% of patients with the CREST syndrome; and in CREST patients the pulmonary hypertension is frequently not associated with interstitial fibrosis. Both plexogenic and nonplexogenic types of pulmonary hypertension may occur in scleroderma and the CREST syndrome patients (Fig. 5.12).

NEUROLOGICAL INVOLVEMENT

Until recently, neurological involvement in scleroderma was considered unusual. The recognized neurological manifestations of scleroderma include peripheral neuropathy and, less commonly, central nervous system, autonomic nervous system, and cranial nerve abnormalities. Lee et al., in 1984, studied neurological involvement prospectively in 125 patients with scleroderma and they were able to identify only four cases of carpal tunnel syndrome, and one each of peripheral neuropathy, trigeminal neuralgia and mononeuritis multiplex. Inclusion of patients with scleroderma myopathy probably contributed to the high incidence (40%) of neurological abnormalities in a more recent retrospective study of 50 scleroderma patients reported by Averbuch-Heller et al. in 1992. Three possible mechanisms may contribute singly or together to the pathogenesis of neurological manifestations in scleroderma and, they are, in descending order of likelihood: fibrosis, a noninflammatory microangiopathy affecting the blood supply of neural tissue, and vasculitis. Biopsies are seldom performed except for ruling out vasculitis in peripheral neuropathy, and vasculitis occurs more commonly in scleroderma associated with another connective tissue disease—the overlap syndrome.

BIBLIOGRAPHY

Abu-Shakra M, Lee P: Mortality in systemic sclerosis: A comparison with the general population. *J Rheumatol* 22:2100–2102, 1995.

Åkesson A, Wollheim FA: Organ manifestations in 100 patients with progressive systemic sclerosis: A comparison between the CREST syndrome and diffuse scleroderma. *Br J Rheumatol* 28:281–286, 1989.

Alusik S, Kovac J, Peregrin J: Large arteries involvement in scleroderma. *Angiology* 41:973–976, 1990.

Altman RD, Medsger TA Jr, Bloch DA, Michel BA: Predictors of survival in systemic sclerosis (scleroderma). *Arthritis Rheum* 34:403–413, 1991.

Anvari A, Graninger W, Schneider B, et al: Cardiac involvement in systemic sclerosis. *Arthritis Rheum* 35:1356–1361, 1992.

Averbuch-Heller L, Steiner I, Abramsky O: Neurologic manifestations of progressive systemic sclerosis. *Arch Neurol* 49:1292–1295, 1992.

Calore EE, Cavaliere MJ, Perez NM, et al: Skeletal muscle pathology in systemic sclerosis. *J Rheumatol* 22:2246–2249, 1995.

Bulkley BH, Ridolfi RC, Salyer WR, Hutchins GM: Myocardial lesions of progressive systemic sclerosis: A cause for cardiac dysfunction. *Circulation* 53:483–490, 1976.

D'Angelo WA, Fries JF, Masi AT, Shulman LE: Pathologic observations in systemic sclerosis (scleroderma): A study of fifty-eight autopsy cases and fifty-eight matched controls. *Am J Med* 46:428–440, 1969.

Donohue JF: Scleroderma and the kidney. *Kidney Int* 41:462–477, 1992.

Eknoyan G, Suki WN: Renal vascular phenomena in systemic sclerosis (scleroderma). *Semin Nephrol* 5:34–45, 1985.

Grishman E, Churg J, Needle MA, Venkataseshan VS (eds): *The Kidney in Collagen-Vascular Diseases.* New York, Raven Press, 1993:121–147.

Herrick AL: Neurological involvement in systemic sclerosis. *Br J Rheumatol* 34:1007–1008, 1995.

Lababidi HMS, Narr FW, Khatib Z: Juvenile progressive systemic sclerosis. Report of five cases. *J Rheumatol* 18:885–888, 1991.

Lee P, Bruni J, Sukenik S: Neurological manifestations in systemic sclerosis (scleroderma). *J Rheumatol* 11:480–483, 1984.

LeRoy EC, Black C, Flieschmajer R, et al: Scleroderma (systemic sclerosis): Classification, subsets and pathogenesis. *J Rheumatol* 15:202–205, 1988.

Lie JT: Pulmonary hypertension in the CREST syndrome: Variant of systemic sclerosis (scleroderma). *Angiology* 40:764–767, 1989.

Lie JT: Rheumatic connective tissue diseases. In Dail DH, Hammar SP (eds); *Pulmonary Pathology,* ed 2. New York, Springer-Verlag, 1994:679–705.

Lomeo RM, Cornella RJ, Schbel SI, Silver RM: Progressive systemic sclerosis sine scleroderma presenting as pulmonary interstitial fibrosis. *Am J Med* 87:525–527, 1989.

Moore HC, Sheehan HL: The kidney of scleroderma. *Lancet* 1:68–70, 1952.

Oddis CV, Eisenbeis CH, Reidbord HE, Steen VD, Medsger TA Jr: Vasculitis in systemic sclerosis: Association with Sjögren's syndrome and the CREST syndrome variant. *J Rheumatol* 14:942–948, 1987.

Oram S, Stokes W: The heart in scleroderma. *Br Heart J* 23:243–259, 1961.

Pisko E, Gallup K, Turner R, et al: Cardiopulmonary manifestations of progressive systemic sclerosis: Associations with circulating immune complexes and fluorescent antinuclear antibodies. *Arthritis Rheum* 22:518–523, 1979.

Rodnan GP, Benedek TG: An historical account of the study of progressive systemic sclerosis (diffuse scleroderma). *Ann Intern Med* 57:305–319, 1962.

Rodnan GP, Schreiner GE, Black RL: Renal involvement in progressive systemic sclerosis (generalized scleroderma). *Am J Med* 23:445–462, 1957.

Silver RM, Miller KS: Lung involvement in systemic sclerosis. *Rheum Dis Clin North Am* 16:199–216, 1990.

Steen VD, Owens GR, Fino GJ, et al: Pulmonary involvement in systemic sclerosis (scleroderma). *Arthritis Rheum* 28:759–767, 1985.

Stupi AM, Steen VD, Owens GR, et al: Pulmonary hypertension in the CREST syndrome variant of systemic sclerosis. *Arthritis Rheum* 29:515–524, 1986.

Tashkin DP, Clement PJ, Wright RS, et al: Interrelationships between pulmonary and extrapulmonary involvement in systemic sclerosis: A longitudinal study. *Chest* 105:489–495, 1994.

Ungerer RG, Tashkin DP, Furst D, et al: Prevalence and clinical correlates of pulmonary arterial hypertension in progressive systemic sclerosis. *Am J Med* 75:65–74, 1983.

Veale DJ, Collidge TA, Belch JJF: Increased prevalence of symptomatic macrovascular disease in systemic sclerosis. *Ann Rheum Dis* 54:853–855, 1995.

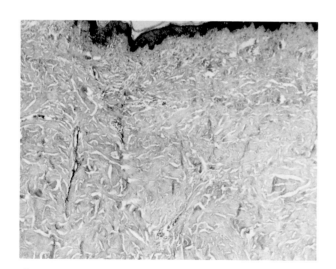

Figure 5.1. Skin biopsy in scleroderma showing thinning of epidermis with loss of rete pegs, and dense fibrosis in the dermis with loss of adnexal structures.

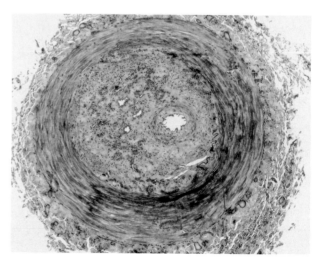

Figure 5.2. Digital artery in scleroderma showing occlusive intimal proliferation with features of an organized thrombus.

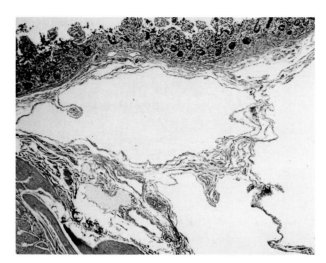

Figure 5.3. Pneumatosis cystoides intestinalis of small bowel in scleroderma.

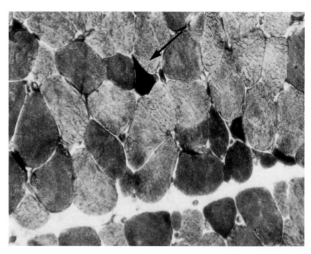

Figure 5.4. Intense histochemical staining of atrophic angulated muscle fiber (*arrow*) expressing neural cell adhesion molecule. (*Courtesy of Dr. E. E. Calore*)

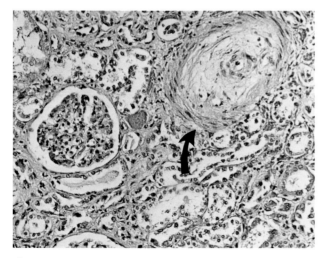

Figure 5.5. Occlusive mucoid intimal proliferation of a renal arteriole (*arrow*) in scleroderma.

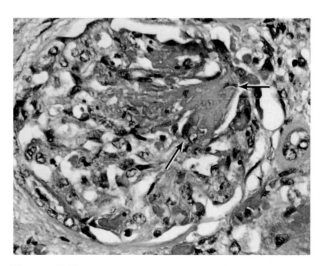

Figure 5.6. Glomerular capillary occlusion with fibrin thrombi (*arrows*) in a scleroderma kidney.

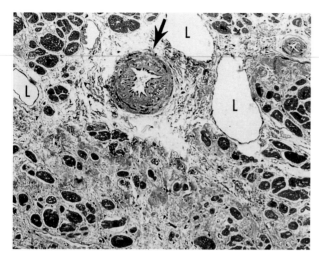

Figure 5.7. Myocardial occlusive small-vessel disease (*arrow*) with dilated lymphatics (*L*) and extensive interstitial fibrosis in scleroderma.

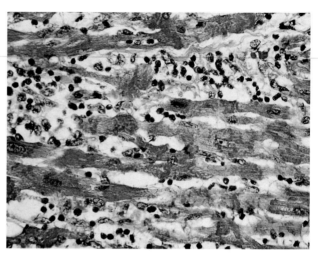

Figure 5.8. A nonspecific myocarditis with myofibrillar degeneration, so-called contraction band necrosis, in scleroderma.

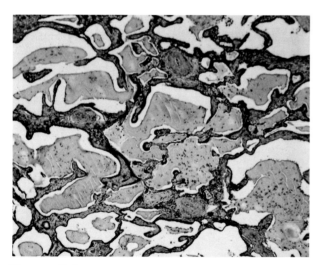

Figure 5.9. Subpleural honey-combing of end-stage pulmonary fibrosis in scleroderma.

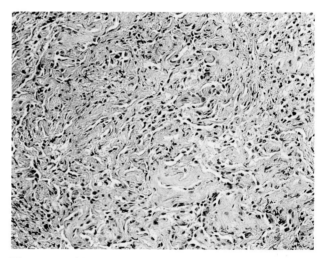

Figure 5.10. Interstitial lung disease in scleroderma, indistinguishable from the idiopathic usual interstitial pneumonitis.

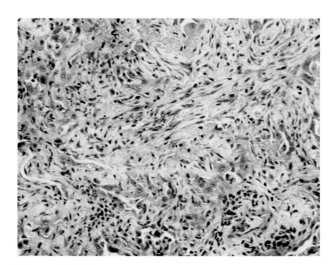

Figure 5.11. Diffuse alveolar damage and bronchiolitis obliterans in scleroderma.

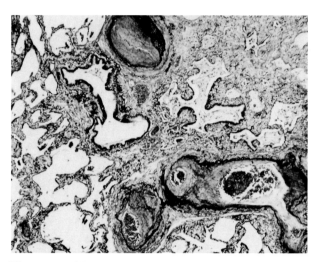

Figure 5.12. Arteriopathy of plexogenic pulmonary hypertension in scleroderma.

6. Dermatopolymyositis

Dermatomyositis and polymyositis are closely related inflammatory myopathies of unknown cause. A characteristic skin rash occurs in the former and not in the latter, but both are in reality a systemic disease often lumped as one clinicopathologic entity and designated as dermatopolymyositis (DPM). Childhood or juvenile dermatomyositis is a distinct subset of DPM with more variable clinical outcome and a systemic vasculopathy as its hallmark.

The term *polymyositis* was first used by Ernst Wagner (1829–1888) in 1887 and, in 1891, Heinrich Unverricht (1858–1912) introduced the name *dermatomyositis* in describing a case. DPM occurs worldwide and has been reported in all races. The disease may develop in a patient of any age, with the highest incidence in the fifth and sixth decades of life and a female:male ratio of 3:2 or 2:1. Cardiac involvement in DPM was first noted by Hermann Oppenheim (1858–1919) in 1899, and the association of DPM with malignancy first became known in 1916. An overlap in clinical features or laboratory findings, or both, of DPM with each of the other classic connective tissue diseases has been recognized since 1939; and the first documentation of interstitial lung disease in DPM appeared a little later, in 1956.

The diagnosis of DPM may be suspected clinically and supported by elevated serum creatinine phosphokinase and aldolase levels and the appropriate electromyographic findings, the latter may help indicate the best sites for muscle biopsy for confirmation. For possible cardiac, pulmonary, and gastrointestinal involvement in DPM, endomyocardial, open lung, and endoscopic biopsy, respectively, is recommended. The central and peripheral nervous system may be affected in DPM. The clinical manifestations of "neurodermatomyositis" include mental confusion, psychosis, delirium, depressed or absent deep tendon reflexes, hyperesthesia and foot drop. The biopsy has no role in the diagnosis of these disorders.

MUSCULOCUTANEOUS AND VASCULAR CHANGES

The skin biopsy findings may be similar to those in patients with scleroderma, with perhaps less prominent epidermal atrophy and dermal fibrosis. A nonspecific lymphomononuclear small-vessel perivascular infiltrate may be observed in the dermis and subcutaneous tissue.

The muscle biopsy findings vary according to the duration of the disease at the time of the biopsy. Biopsy confirmation of the clinical diagnosis of DPM may be inconclusive if symptoms have been present for only a short time. After the disease becomes established, the definite myopathic changes and inflammatory infiltrates tend to be concentrated at the periphery of the muscle fascicle (Fig. 6.1). The late changes are characterized by atrophy, and degeneration and regeneration of muscle fibers with infiltrate of macrophages (Fig. 6.2).

Small-vessel vasculitis occurs more commonly in juvenile DPM than in adults, and it may be a polyarteritis-type necrotizing vasculitis (Fig. 6.3) or a non-necrotizing lymphocytic vasculitis (Fig. 6.4) of the skeletal muscle, or, less frequently, in visceral organs.

RENAL DISEASE

The kidneys are generally spared in DPM, but the reported incidence of abnormal urinalysis and renal function tests varies from 0 to 70% of patients and acute myoglobulinuric renal failure secondary to rhabdomyolysis certainly may develop in a few patients.

All known renal parenchymal lesions in DPM have been preceded clinically by significant urinary abnormalities and, sometimes, by decreased creatinine clearance. Focal or diffuse mesangial proliferative glomerulonephritis (Fig. 6.5) or nonspecific mesangial changes are observed in most reported cases, and immunofluorescence microscopy have revealed focal or diffuse deposits of immunoglobulin and complement in some cases.

CARDIAC INVOLVEMENT

Cardiac symptoms as presenting complaints are clinically apparent in only 10–15% of DPM patients, although functional cardiac abnormalities may be detected by noninvasive means in over 70%, principally nonspecific electrocardiographic changes. Myocardial small vessel occlusive disease with interstitial fibrosis (Fig. 6.6) or coronary vasculitis (Fig. 6.7), and a nonspecific myocarditis (Fig. 6.8) have been detected in up to 30% of patients, previously only at autopsy but now in endomyocardial biopsies. These morphologic abnormalities may be observed in both the contractile and conduction myocardium, and their presence correlates with the development of arrhythmia and cardiac failure in DPM patients.

PULMONARY MANIFESTATIONS

Pulmonary involvement in DPM was first described by Mills and Matthews as recently as 1956; the reported prevalence rate varies from 0 to 64% but most probably in the 10–15% range. Earlier investigators described three types of pulmonary involvement: (1) ventilatory insufficiency due to respiratory muscle weakness; (2) aspiration pneumonia; and (3) usual interstitial pneumonitis (Fig. 6.9). More recent studies emphasize the occurrence of diffuse alveolar damage and bronchiolitis obliterans (Fig. 6.10) and, less commonly, respiratory vasculitis (Fig. 6.11) and pulmonary hypertension (Fig. 6.12).

The prognosis of DPM patients with pulmonary involvement is generally unfavorable; the case fatality rate for those with biopsy proven inflammatory myopathy and interstitial lung disease is >60% over a 2-year period. Clinically, the interstitial lung disease may precede evidence of inflammatory myopathy in about one-third of cases, and patients with diffuse alveolar damage or pulmonary vascular disease have a uniformly poor prognosis.

BIBLIOGRAPHY

Ansell BM: Juvenile dermatomyositis. In Ansell BM, Bacon PA, Lie JT, Yazici H (eds): *The Vasculitides, Science and Practice.* London, Chapman & Hall, 1996:377–383.

Ansura EL, Greenberg AS: Adverse impact of interstitial pulmonary fibrosis on prognosis in polymyositis and dermatomyositis. *Semin Arthritis Rheum* 18:29–37, 1988.

Askari AD, Huettner TL: Cardiac abnormalities in polymyositis/dermatomyositis. *Semin Arthritis Rheum* 12: 208–219, 1982.

Banker BQ, Victor M: Dermatomyositis (systemic angiopathy) of childhood. *Medicine* 45:261–289, 1966.

Bohan A, Peters JB: Polymyositis and dermatomyositis. *N Engl J Med* 292:344–347 and 403–407, 1975.

Bunch TW, Tancredi RG, Lie JT: Pulmonary hypertension in polymyositis. *Chest* 79:105–107, 1981.

Crowe WE, Bove KE, Levinson JE, Hilton PK: Clinical and pathogenetic implications of histopathology in childhood polydermatomyositis. *Arthritis Rheum* 25: 126–139, 1982.

Denbow CE, Lie JT, Tancredi RG, Bunch TW: Cardiac involvement in polymyositis: A clinicopathologic study of 20 autopsied patients. *Arthritis Rheum* 22: 1088–1092, 1979.

Dickey BF, Myers AR: Pulmonary disease in polymyositis/dermatomyositis. *Semin Arthritis Rheum* 13:60–76, 1984.

Gardner DG: *Pathological Basis of the Connective Tissue Diseases.* Philadelphia, Lea & Febiger, 1992: 675–693.

Grishman E, Churg, Needle MA, Venkataseshan VS (eds): *The Kidney in Collagen-Vascular Diseases.* New York, Raven Press., 1993:189–211.

Haupt HM, Hutchins GM: The heart and cardiac conduction system in polymyositis-dermatomyositis: A clinicopathologic study of 16 autopsied patients. *Am J Cardiol* 50:998–1006, 1982.

Kankeleit H: Über primäre nichteitrige Polymyositis. *Dtsch Arch klin Med* 120:335–349, 1916.

Lakhanpal S, Bunch TW, Ilstrup DM, Melton LJ III: Polymyositis-dermatomyositis and malignant lesions: Does an association exist? *Mayo Clin Proc* 61:645–653, 1986.

Lakhanpal S, Lie JT, Conn DL, Martin WJ II: Pulmonary disease in polymyositis-dermatomyositis: A clinicopathological analysis of 65 autopsy cases. *Ann Rheum Dis* 46:23–29, 1987.

Lie JT: Rheumatic connective tissue diseases. In Dail DH, Hammar SP (eds): *Pulmonary Pathology,* ed 2. New York, Springer-Verlag, 1994:679–705.

Mills ES, Matthews WH: Interstitial pneumonitis in dermatomyositis. *JAMA* 160:1467–1470, 1956.

Oppenheim H: Zur Dermatomyositis. *Berl klin Wchnschr* 36:805–807, 1899.

Plotz PH, Dalakas M, Leff RL, et al: Current concepts in the idiopathic inflammatory myopathies: Polymyositis, dermatomyositis, and related disorders. *Ann Intern Med* 111:143–157, 1989.

Rechavia E, Rotenberg Z, Fuchs J, Strasberg B: Polymyositis heart disease. *Chest* 88:309–311, 1985.

Strongwater SL, Annesley T, Schnitzer TJ: Myocardial involvement in polymyositis. *J Rheumatol* 10:459–463, 1983.

Sullivan DB, Cassidy JT, Petty RE: Dermatomyositis in the pediatric patient. *Arthritis Rheum* 20:327–331, 1977.

Takizawa H, Shiga J, Moroi Y, et al: Interstitial lung disease in dermatomyositis: Clinicopathological study. *J Rheumatol* 14:102–107, 1987.

Tazelaar HD, Viggiano RW, Pickersgill J, Colby TV: Interstitial lung disease in polymyositis and dermatomyositis: Clinical features and prognosis as correlated with histologic findings. *Am Rev Respir Dis* 141: 727–733, 1990.

Unvericht H: Dermatomyositis acuta. *Deutsche med Wchnschr* 17:41–44, 1891.

Wagner E: Ein Fall von acuter polymyositis. *Deutsche Arch klin Med* 40:241–266, 1887.

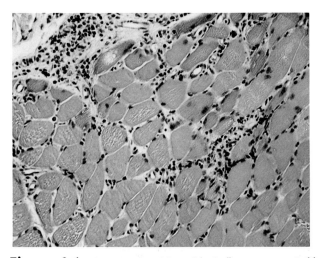

Figure 6.1. Acute myositis with inflammatory infiltrates at the periphery of muscle fascicle.

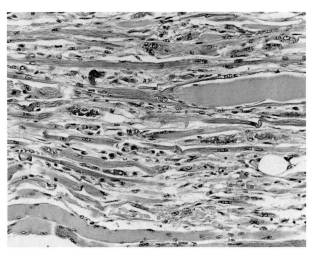

Figure 6.2. Atrophy, and degeneration and regeneration of muscle fibers with infiltrate of macrophages in more chronic phase of polymyositis.

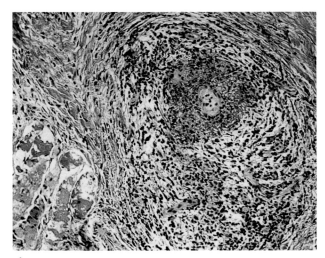

Figure 6.3. Necrotizing vasculitis in a muscle biopsy of juvenile dermatomyositis.

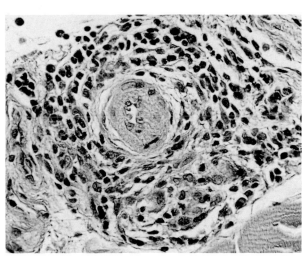

Figure 6.4. A non-necrotizing lymphocytic myositis in dermatopolymyositis.

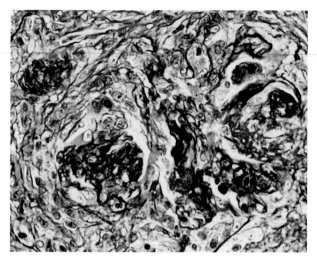

Figure 6.5. Silver methanamine stain renal biopsy section with diffuse mesangial proliferative glomerulonephritis in dermatopolymyositis.

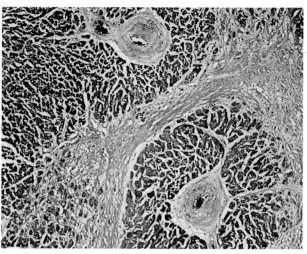

Figure 6.6. Endomyocardial biopsy revealing intramyocardial small-vessel occlusive disease and interstitial fibrosis in dermatopolymyositis.

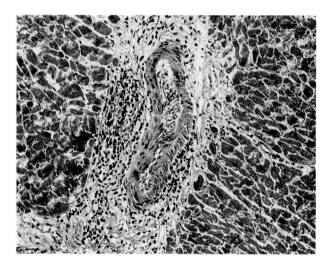

Figure 6.7. Endomyocardial biopsy revealing intramyocardial coronary vasculitis.

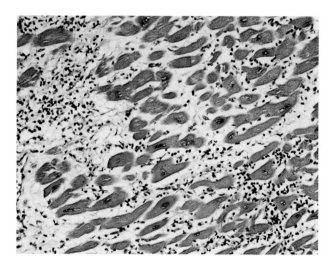

Figure 6.8. A nonspecific myocarditis diagnosed by endomyocardial biopsy.

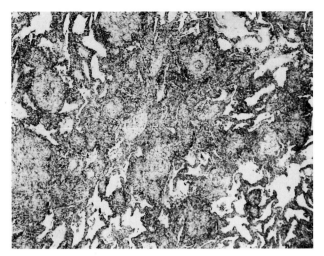

Figure 6.9. Usual interstitial pneumonitis with pulmonary vasculitis in dermatopolymyositis.

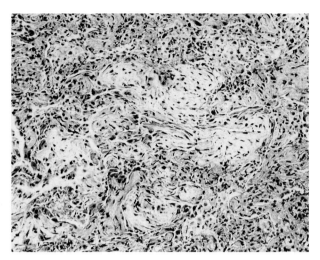

Figure 6.10. Sclerosing alveolitis-bronchiolitis obliterans in dermatopolymyositis.

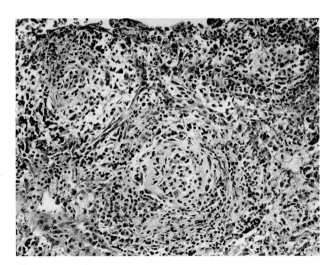

Figure 6.11. Pulmonary vasculitis with predominantly a lymphoplasmacytic infiltrate in a dermatopolymyositis lung biopsy.

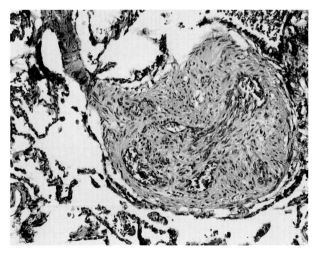

Figure 6.12. Plexiform arteriopathy of pulmonary hypertension in dermatopolymyositis.

7. Sjögren's Syndrome

The clinical entity originally known as *keratoconjunctivitis sicca* (dry eyes) *and xerostomia* (dry mouth) was first described at a meeting of the Clinical Society of London by William Hadden in 1888. It was later studied more extensively by the Swedish ophthalmologist Henrik Samuel Conrad Sjögren who, in 1933, published his first monograph on the disorder that now becomes widely known as Sjögren's syndrome (SJS).

SJS is a chronic and slowly progressive inflammatory exocrinopathy of unknown cause, commonly occurs in middle-aged women but is known to affect men and women of all ages. The typical clinical presentation of SJS is the glandular manifestations of the syndrome keratoconjunctivitis sicca and xerostomia; extraglandular systemic manifestations are diverse (Table 7.1), occurring in about one-half of primary SJS, 5 to 10 years after the diagnosis.

Next to rheumatoid arthritis, SJS is the second most common autoimmune rheumatic disorder. When SJS is not associated with other connective tissue diseases, the syndrome is designated as *primary*, while *secondary* SJS refers to the syndrome coexisting with a wide variety of other autoimmune disorders that include rheumatoid arthritis, systemic lupus erythematosus, scleroderma, dermatopolymyositis, mixed connective tissue disease, primary biliary cirrhosis, chronic active hepatitis, thyroiditis, vasculitis, mixed cryoglobulinemia, and hypergammaglobulinemic purpura. Thus, diagnosis on clinical grounds alone is difficult.

During the past three decades, several different sets of diagnostic criteria for SJS have been proposed and the most recent one was the 1993 Classification Criteria (Table 7.2) developed by the European Community Study Group with data from 26 centers in 12 countries, comprising a total of 486 patients with primary SJS, 201 with secondary SJS, 113 with connective tissue diseases unassociated with SJS, and 373 age- and sex-matched controls.

DIAGNOSIS OF SJÖGREN'S SYNDROME

Diagnosis of SJS is usually initiated by a combination of concordant patient's clinical history, subjective symptoms, bedside and laboratory objective findings; and selective biopsies are undertaken only after the results of clinical and laboratory evaluations suggest SJS as the disease in question.

Hematologically, a mild normocytic and normochromic anemia occurs in about 25% of patients, leukopenia but with a relative eosinophilia (5 to 7% of the total leukocyte count) in 25%, and a Westergren erythrocyte sedimentation rate of >30 mm/hr in more than 90%. A high proportion of SJS patients (±50%) have demonstrable circulating immune complexes, hypocomplementemia, cryoglobulinemia, and macroglobulinemia. The peripheral blood T-lymphocytes are decreased in about one-third of patients, and abnormalities of T-cell function are detectable particularly in patients with SJS related lymphoproliferative disorders.

Autoantibodies are common in SJS: rheumatoid factor >1:320 in 75 to 90% of patients; antinuclear antibodies >1:320 in 50 to 75% of patients; antibodies to nucleoprotein antigens SS-A (Ro) and SS-B (La) in >60% of patients; and presence of multiple organ-specific autoantibodies (against gastric parietal, thyroid microsomal, thyroglobulin, mitochondrial, smooth muscle, and salivary duct antigens) in 25 to 30%.

SALIVARY AND LACRIMAL GLAND BIOPSIES

The exocrine glandular component of SJS is characterized by lymphocytic infiltration of the lacrimal glands, and of the major and minor salivary glands, leading to the classic symptoms of keratoconjunctivitis (dry eyes)and xerostomia (dry mouth), respectively. Labial salivary gland (LSG) as the preferable biopsy site has been used since 1972, and the desired tissue is obtained through a linear incision of the lower labial mucosa between the midline and the commissure. This method provides sufficient number of glands for histological examination, with low risk of sensory nerve damage and a nondisfiguring rapid wound healing.

LSG biopsy is done under the assumption that the findings reflect changes that would have been observed also in the major salivary glands. Biopsy of the parotid gland is usually considered a more risky procedure, but there have been comparative studies suggesting that parotid gland biopsy has greater sensitivity for SJS than LSG biopsy. Lacrimal gland biopsy also offers greater sensitivity in the diagnosis of SJS but concerns with complications affecting lacrimation, bleeding, and fistula formation have prevented its widespread use.

A standardized semiquantitative grading system for LSG biopsies in SJS was devised by Chisholm and Mason in 1968, and it received universal acceptance and has been included in the classification criteria for SJS (Table 7.2). According to the number of lympho-

Table 7.1 Estimated Frequency of Clinical Manifestations of Sjögren's Syndrome*

Clinical Manifestations	Percent
Sicca complex (dry eyes and dry mouth)	90
Arthralgia and arthritis	60
Raynaud's phenomenon	35
Lymphadenopathy	15
Lung involvement	15
Vasculitis	10
Renal involvement	10
Gastrointestinal or hepatic involvement	10
Lymphoma	5
Peripheral neuropathy	5
Myositis	3
Splenomegaly	2

*Modified from Schumacher HR, Klippel JH, Koopman (eds): *Primer on Rheumatic Diseases, ed 10.* Atlanta, The Arthritis Foundation, 1993:133.

Table 7.2 Preliminary Classification Criteria of Sjögren's Syndrome Developed By The European Community Study Group*

A. Ocular symptoms (at least one present)
   1. Daily, persistent, troublesome dry eyes for more than 3 months
   2. Recurrent sensation of sand or gravel in the eyes
   3. Use of tear substitute more than 3 times a day
B. Oral symptoms (at least one present)
   1. Daily feeling of dry mouth for at least 3 months
   2. Recurrent feeling of swollen salivary glands as adult
   3. Drinking liquid to aid in washing down dry foods
C. Objective evidence of dry eyes (at least one present)
   1. Schirmer test
   2. Rose Bengal test
   3. Lacrimal gland biopsy with focus score >1
D. Objective evidence of salivary gland involvement (at least one present)
   1. Salivary gland scintigraphy
   2. Parotid gland sialography
   3. Unstimulated whole sialometry (<1.5 mL per 15 minutes)
   4. Salivary gland biopsy with focus score >1
E. Laboratory abnormality (at least one present)
   1. IgM rheumatoid factor >1:320
   2. Antinuclear antibody >1:320
   3. Anti SS-A (Ro) or anti SS-B (La) antibodies

*Modified from Vitali C, et al. *Arthritis Rheum* 1993;36:340–347 and Fox RI, Saito I. *Rheum Dis Clin North Am* 1994;20:391–407.

cytes present per 4 mm^2 of salivary gland tissue, a LSG biopsy is graded as "0" for absence of infiltrate, as "1" for slight infiltrate, as "2" for moderate infiltrate but less than one "focus," as "3" for one "focus," and as "4" for more than one "focus;" a "focus" is defined as an aggregate of 50 or more lymphocytes and histiocytes per 4 mm^2 of gland tissue.

A "focus" may appear as diffuse infiltrate of the glandular component (Fig. 7.1) or of the ductular component (Fig. 7.2) in a LSG biopsy. Grade 4 LSG biopsies are seen in the majority of primary (about 65%) and secondary (about 80%) SJS patients. The specific feature of ductal or ductular wall with infiltrating lymphocytes (Fig. 7.3) has not been accorded with the importance that it justifies, because it is observed in >60% of primary SJS and in only <10% of secondary SJS or focal sialadenitis. LSG is also useful for the biopsy diagnosis of pseudolymphoma or lymphoma associated with SJS (Fig. 7.4).

INFLAMMATORY VASCULAR DISEASE

Pulmonary, gastrointestinal, cerebral, and cutaneous involvements are extraglandular manifestations of SJS that may be an important source of morbidity and mortality, and small-vessel vasculitis is often implicated as the common underlying cause.

There is a close association between the presence of antibodies to SS-A (Ro) and the occurrence of vasculitis in SJS. The reported incidence of vasculitis in SJS patients ranges from 13 to 33%, and cutaneous vasculitis is the most common variety. According to some investigators, two histologic types of vasculitis occur in SJS: vasculitis with mononuclear infiltrate, or a nonnecrotizing (Fig. 7.5); and vasculitis with neutrophilic infiltrate, or a necrotizing vasculitis (Fig. 7.6). A third type, the granulomatous vasculitis (Fig. 7.7) has been described recently. Other investigators classify vasculitis in SJS into four categories: (1) acute necrotizing vasculitis; (2) leukocytoclastic vasculitis; (3) lymphocytic vasculitis; and (4) endarteritis obliterans. This difference of opinions is more apparent than real, because a neutrophilic infiltrate characterizes both necrotizing vasculitis and leukocytoclastic vasculitis, and "endarteritis obliterans" is a descriptive term for healed vasculitis with either neutrophilic or lymphocytic infiltrate in its acute phase.

NEUROMUSCULAR INVOLVEMENT

Clinically, peripheral neuropathy and central nervous system disease are not uncommon in patients with primary or secondary SJS but their incidence rates have not been determined. In reported retrospective series of cases, most of the neurological symptoms were mild and when found in patients with secondary SJS were characteristic of the associated autoimmune diseases such as rheumatoid arthritis and systemic lupus erythematosus. There appeared to be no significant association between the frequency of either vasculitis or any autoantibodies and the presence of neurologic disease, but there was a significant association between vasculitis and the presence of antibodies to extractable nuclear antigens.

Late-onset inflammatory myopathy has been observed infrequently in SJS patients, and only one large series of myositis in SJS has been published, that of Denco et al. in 1969. The muscle biopsy findings include necrosis, phagocytosis, degeneration and regeneration of muscle fibers with an interstitial lymphocytic infiltrate (Fig. 7.8).

PULMONARY MANIFESTATIONS

Pulmonary manifestations of SJS occur in 10 to 15% of patients, and include pleuritis, diffuse interstitial fibrosis, alveolitis and bronchiolitis obliterans, lymphocytic interstitial pneumonitis (LIP), and lymphoma, of which LIP is probably the most common (Fig. 7.9). It has been suggested that LIP is the consequence of SJS while diffuse interstitial fibrosis is related to the associated connective tissue disease. Pulmonary vasculitis (Fig. 7.10) and pulmonary hypertension (Fig. 7.11) are seldom observed, and mostly in women.

RENAL DISEASE

Renal disease probably occurs more often than it is recognized. The most common abnormal renal biopsy finding in SJS is interstitial nephritis (Fig. 7.12) which may be subclinical. The majority of the infiltrating lymphocytes in the kidney, as they are in salivary glands, have been found to be activated helper/inducer T-lymphocytes. The pathogenesis of interstitial nephritis in SJS is not well understood; immune complex deposits, cell-mediated immunity, and hypergammaglobulinemia have all been implicated as possible etiologic factors.

BIBLIOGRAPHY

Alexander E: Central nervous system disease in Sjögren's syndrome. *Rheum Dis Clin North Am* 18:637–672, 1992.

Alexander EL, Arnett FC, Provost TT, Stevens MB: Sjögren's syndrome: Association of anti Ro (SS-A) antibodies with vasculitis. *Ann Intern Med* 98:155–159, 1983.

Alexander EL, Provost TT: Cutaneous manifestations of primary Sjögren's syndrome: A reflection of vasculitis and association with anti Ro (SS-A) antibodies. *J Invest Dermatol* 80:386–391, 1983.

Binder A, Snaith ML, Isenberg D: Sjögren's syndrome: A study of its neurological complications. *Br J Rheumatol* 27:275–280, 1988.

Bloch KJ, Buchanan WW, Wohl MJ, Bunim JJ: Sjögren's syndrome: A clinical, pathological, and serological study of sixty-two cases. *Medicine* 44:187–231, 1965.

Chisholm DM, Mason DK: Labial salivary gland biopsy in Sjögren's disease. *J Clin Pathol* 21:656–660, 1968.

Chisholm DM, Waterhouse JP, Mason DK: Lymphocytic sialadenitis in the major and minor glands: A correlation in postmortem subjects. *J Clin Pathol* 23:690–694, 1970.

Constantopoulos SH, Tsianos EV, Moutsopoulos HM: Pulmonary and gastrointestinal manifestations of Sjögren's syndrome. *Rheum Dis Clin North Am* 18:617–635, 1992.

Daniels TE: Labial salivary gland biopsy in Sjögren's syndrome: Assessment as a diagnostic criterion in 362 suspected cases. *Arthritis Rheum* 27:147–156, 1984.

Daniels TE: Salivary histopathology in diagnosis of Sjögren's syndrome. *Scand J Rheumatol (Suppl)* 61:36–43, 1986.

Daniels TE, Whitcher JP: Association of patterns of labial salivary gland inflammation with keratoconjunctivitis sicca: Analysis of 618 patients with suspected Sjögren's syndrome. *Arthritis Rheum* 37:869–877, 1994.

Eneström S, Denneberg T, Eriksson P: Histopathology of

renal biopsies with correlation to clinical findings in primary Sjögren's syndrome. *Clin Exp Rheumatol* 13: 697–703, 1995.

Ferreiro JE, Robalino BD, Saldana MJ: Primary Sjögren's syndrome with diffuse cerebral vasculitis and lymphocytic interstitial pneumonitis. *Am J Med* 82: 1227–1232, 1987.

Fox RI, Howell FV, Bone RC, Michelson P: Primary Sjögren's syndrome: Clinical and immunopathologic features. *Semin Arthritis Rheum* 14:77–105, 1984.

Fox RI, Robinson CA, Curd JG, Kozin F, Howell FV: Sjögren's syndrome: Proposed criteria for classification. *Arthritis Rheum* 29:577–586, 1986.

Fox RI, Saito I: Criteria for diagnosis of Sjögren's syndrome. *Rheum Dis Clin North Am* 20:291–407, 1994.

Grishman E, Churg J, Needle MA, Venkataseshan VS: *The Kidney in Collagen-Vascular Diseases.* New York, Raven Press 1993:179–187.

Hansen LA, Prakash UBS, Colby TV: Pulmonary lymphoma in Sjögren's syndrome. *Mayo Clin Proc* 64: 920–931, 1989.

Kruize AA, Hené RJ, van der Heide A, et al: Long-term followup of patients with Sjögren's syndrome. *Arthritis Rheum* 39:297–303, 1996.

Leroy J-P, Pennec Y-L, Letoux G, Youinou P: Lymphocytic infiltration of salivary ducts: A histopathologic lesion specific for primary Sjögren's syndrome. *Arthritis Rheum* 35:481, 1992.

Lie JT: Rheumatic connective tissue diseases. In Dail DH, Hammar SP (eds): *Pulmonary Pathology,* ed 2. New York, Springer-Verlag, 1994:679–705

Lie JT: Isolated necrotizing and granulomatous vasculitis causing ischemic bowel disease in primary Sjögren's syndrome. *J Rheumatol* 22:2375–2377, 1995.

Molina R, Provost TT, Alexander EL: Two types of inflammatory vascular disease in Sjögren's syndrome: Differential association with seroactivity to rheumatoid factor and antibodies to Ro (SS-A) and with hypocomplementemia. *Arthritis Rheum* 28: 1251–1258, 1985.

Molina R, Provost TT, Alexander EL: Peripheral inflammatory vascular disease in Sjögren's syndrome: Association with nervous system complications. *Arthritis Rheum* 28:1341–1347, 1985.

Oxholm P, Asmussen K, Axéll T, et al: Sjögren's

syndrome: Terminology. *Clin Exp Rheumatol* 13: 693–696, 1995.

Peyronnard J-M, Charron L, Beaudet F, Couture F: Vasculitic neuropathy in rheumatoid disease and Sjögren's syndrome. *Neurology* 32:839–845, 1982.

Provost TT, Watson R: Cutaneous manifestations of Sjögren's syndrome. *Rheum Dis Clin North Am* 18: 609–616, 1992.

Rayadurg J, Koch AE: Renal insufficiency from interstitial nephritis in primary Sjögren's syndrome. *J Rheumatol* 17:1714–1718, 1990.

Sato T, Matsubara O, Tanaka Y, Kasuga T: Association of Sjögren's syndrome with pulmonary hypertension: Report of two cases and review of the literature. *Hum Pathol* 24:199–205, 1993.

Schiødt M, Thorn J: Criteria for the salivary component of Sjögren's syndrome: A review. *Clin Exp Rheumatol* 7:119–122, 1989.

Segerberg-Konttinen M: A postmortem study of focal adenitis in salivary and lacrimal glands. *J Autoimmunity* 2:553–558, 1989.

Shah F, Rapini RP, Arnett FC, Warner NB, Smith CA: Association of labial salivary gland histopathology with clinical and serologic features of connective tissue diseases. *Arthritis Rheum* 33:1682–1697, 1990.

Talal N: Sjögren's syndrome: Historical overview and clinical spectrum of disease. *Rheum Dis Clin North Am* 18:507–515, 1992.

Tsokos M, Lazarou SA, Moutsopoulos HM: Vasculitis in primary Sjögren's syndrome: Histologic classification and clinical presentation. *Am J Clin Pathol* 88: 26–31, 1987.

Tsubota K, Xu K-P, Fujihara T, et al: Decreased reflex tearing is associated with lymphocytic infiltration in lacrimal glands. *J Rheumatol* 23:313–320, 1996.

Vitali C, Bombardieri S, Moutsopoulos HM, et al: Preliminary criteria for the classification of Sjögren's syndrome. *Arthritis Rheum* 36:340–347, 1993

Wise CM, Agudelo CA, Semble EL, Stump TE, Woodruff RD: Comparison of parotid and minor salivary gland biopsy specimens in the diagnosis of Sjögren's syndrome. *Arthritis Rheum* 31:662–666, 1988.

Wise CM, Woodruff RD: Minor salivary gland biopsies in patients investigated for primary Sjögren's syndrome: A review of 187 patients. *J Rheumatol* 20: 1515–1518, 1993.

Xu K-P, Katagiri S, Takeuchi T, Tsubota K: Biopsy of labial salivary glands and lacrimal glands in the diagnosis of Sjögren's syndrome. *J Rheumatol* 23:76–82, 1996.

Zutniga-Montes LR, Gonzalez-Buritica H: Leg ulcer in a patient with primary Sjögren's syndrome. *Arthritis Rheum* 37:1335–1337, 1994.

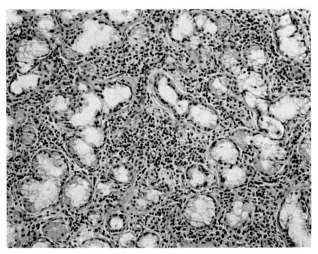

Figure 7.1. Diffuse infiltrate of glandular component of salivary gland with >50 lymphocytes per 4 mm² gland tissue.

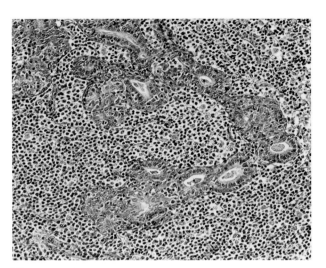

Figure 7.2. Diffuse infiltrate of ductular component of salivary gland with >50 lymphocytes per 4 mm² gland tissue.

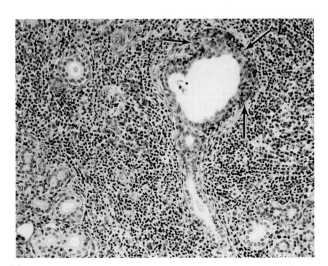

Figure 7.3. Salivary gland ductal wall infiltrated by lymphocytes (*arrows*).

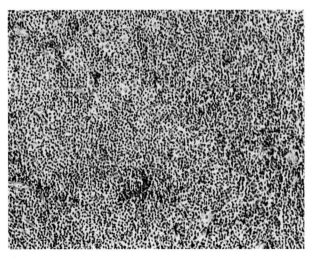

Figure 7.4. Low-grade lymphocytic lymphoma in a salivary gland biopsy.

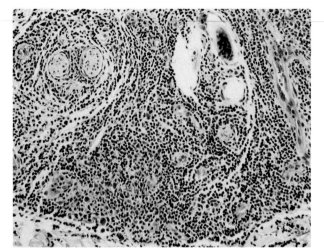

Figure 7.5. A typical cutaneous lymphocytic vasculitis in Sjögren's syndrome.

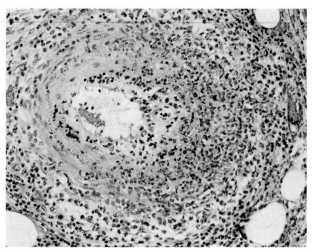

Figure 7.6. A typical visceral neutrophilic necrotizing vasculitis in Sjögren's syndrome.

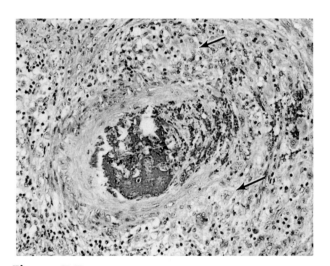

Figure 7.7. A rare visceral granulomatous vasculitis with giant cells (*arrows*) in primary Sjögren's syndrome.

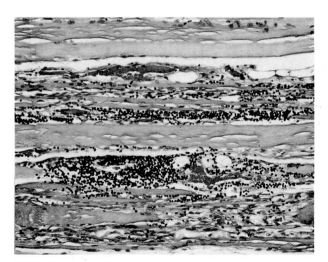

Figure 7.8. Chronic-phase myositis with lymphocytic infiltrate in Sjögren's syndrome.

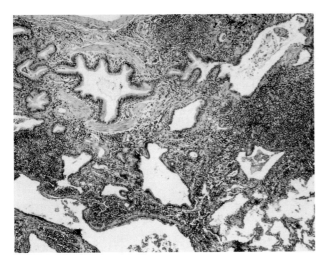

Figure 7.9. Lymphocytic interstitial pneumonitis in Sjögren's syndrome.

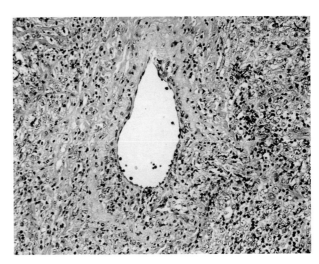

Figure 7.10. Pulmonary vasculitis in Sjögren's syndrome.

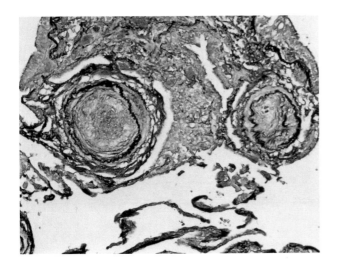

Figure 7.11. Plexiform arteriopathy of pulmonary hypertension in Sjögren's syndrome.

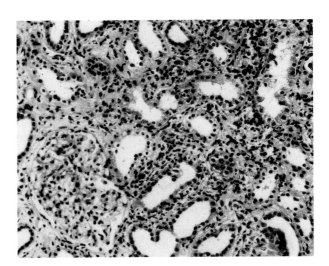

Figure 7.12. Interstitial nephritis with prominent lymphocytic infiltrate in Sjögren's syndrome. (*Courtesy of Dr. Jacob Churg*)

8. Relapsing Polychondritis

Relapsing polychondritis is an uncommon autoimmune disorder manifested by episodic and progressive inflammation and destruction of both articular and nonarticular cartilage. The disorder was originally described as "polychondropathia" in 1923 by Jaksch-Wartenhorst; in 1958 Bean et al. suggested the term "chronic atrophic polychondritis" in a case report and a review of eight previous cases; and the now widely accepted name "relapsing polychondritis" was first used by Pearson et al. two years later.

Relapsing polychondritis is a systemic disease (Table 8.1). Over 30% of patients may have an associated autoimmune or hematologic disorder, including systemic lupus erythematosus, systemic sclerosis, Behçet's disease, Sjögren's syndrome, systemic vasculitis, rheumatoid arthritis, spondylarthropathies, ulcerative colitis, psoriasis vulgaris, autoimmune thyroiditis, diabetes mellitus, pernicious anemia, and dysmyelopoietic syndromes; clinically some of which may antedate relapsing polychondritis by months to years.

To date, about 450 to 500 cases of relapsing polychondritis worldwide have been documented in the literature. The disease occurs in all age groups, the male:female ratio of the patients is close to unity, and the five-year survival is about 75%. Death has usually been attributed to airway obstruction or pulmonary infection, or both, and to cardiovascular complications that include myocarditis, valvular heart disease, aortitis, arterial aneurysmal disease and vasculitis.

Although the etiology of relapsing polychondritis remains unknown, individual susceptibility is associated with a significantly higher frequency of HLA-DR4 as compared with that in normal controls, but there is no known predominance of any DR4 subtype. The presence of antibodies to type II and other collagens in the serum of patients suggests that responses by the body's immune system to the cartilage and other types of collagen participate in the pathogenesis of the disease.

CLINICAL DIAGNOSIS

Clinical studies have established diagnostic criteria for relapsing polychondritis on an empirical basis. McAdam et al. (1976), Damiani and Levine (1979), and Isaak et al. (1986) proposed that a diagnosis requires three or more of the following clinical criteria, or one clinical feature together with a compatible biopsy, or chondritis in two or more separate anatomical sites together with a favorable therapeutic response to corticosteroids. The major clinical criteria are: (1) recurrent auricular chondritis; (2) nonerosive, seronegative inflammatory polyarthritis; (3) nasal chondritis; (4) ocular inflammation (conjunctivitis, keratitis, scleritis/episcleritis, uveitis); (5) respiratory tract chondritis (laryngeal and/or tracheal cartilages); (6) cochlear or vestibular dysfunction (neurosensory hearing loss, tinnitus, and/or vertigo).

BIOPSY DIAGNOSIS

A biopsy is often considered unnecessary when the clinical diagnosis of relapsing polychondritis may be obvious in established cases. However, if the history is recent or scanty and the clinical picture unclear or confusing, a biopsy is essential for the diagnosis.

Chondritis

At the height of the inflammatory process, biopsy of an affected otorhinolaryngeal cartilage will show an inflammatory infiltrate consisting of predominantly CD4-positive lymphocytes at the fibrocartilaginous junction in a vascularized stroma, but rarely necrosis of the cartilage or a true vasculitis (Figs. 8.1 and 8.2).

Cardiovascular Involvement

Cardiovascular involvement, occurring in up to 10% of the patients, is an important systemic manifestation of relapsing polychondritis. Biopsy procedures are determined by the evidence of involvement and accessibility of tissue samples. Myocarditis may manifest as heart failure of unknown cause, arrhythmia, or heart block, and be diagnosed with an endomyocardial biopsy (Fig. 8.3). Autoimmune valvulitis causing cusp rupture and valvular dysfunction has been diagnosed unexpectedly on tissue obtained at valve replacement surgery for aortic and/or mitral insufficiency (Fig. 8.4). Aortitis and/or multiple arterial aneurysms may also be manifestations of relapsing polychondritis but the diagnosis cannot be confirmed without adequate tissue obtained at the time of surgical intervention. On the other hand, leukocytoclastic vasculitis, although nonspecific, is readily diagnosed in a skin biopsy (Fig. 8.5). The more inaccessible visceral biopsies are needed for the diagnosis of the polyarteritis-type small or medium-sized vessel disease in relapsing polychondritis.

Table 8.1 Clinical Manifestations of Relapsing Polychondritis*

Clinical Manifestation	Initial (%)	Final (%)
Auricular chondritis	40	85
Nasal chondritis	20	50
Hearing loss	10	30
Ocular disease	20	50
Laryngotracheal chondritis	25	50
Laryngotracheal stricture	15	25
Nonerosive arthritis	35	50
Systemic vasculitis	5	10
Valvular heart disease	0	5

*Modified from Isaak et al: *Ophthalmology* 93: 681–689, 1986

Renal Involvement

The incidence of renal involvement in relapsing polychondritis is unknown but significant renal disease has been observed in about 10% of the reported cases. Renal disease may occur concomitantly or a few months to years after the initial diagnosis of relapsing polychondritis. Patients with renal involvement tend to be older and more commonly have arthritis or a systemic vasculitis. The spectrum of renal disease seen in a biopsy includes focal segmental necrotizing glomerulonephritis (Fig. 8.6), which is most common, followed by proliferative mesangial glomerulonephritis, crescenteric glomerulonephritis, focal or global glomerulosclerosis, and interstitial nephritis, none of which is specific for or diagnostic of relapsing polychondritis. By immunofluorescence microscopy, a variety of immunoglobulins and complements in a granular pattern have been observed in the glomerular mesangium. Evidence of necrotizing renal arteritis or healed vasculitic lesions of the renal artery has been described only in autopsy specimens.

BIBLIOGRAPHY

Arkin CR, Masi AT: Relapsing polychondritis: Review of current status and case report. *Semin Arthritis Rheum* 5:41–52, 1975.

Alsalameh S, Mollenhauer J, Scheuplein F, et al: Preferential cellular and humoral immune reactivities to native and denatured collagen types IX and XI in a patient with fatal relapsing polychondritis. *J Rheumatol* 20:1419–1424, 1993.

Bean WB, Drevets CC, Chapman JS: Chronic atrophic polychondritis. *Medicine* 37:353–363, 1958.

Botey A, Navasa M, del Olmo A, et al: Relapsing polychondritis with segmental necrotizing glomerulonephritis. *Am J Nephrol* 4:375–378, 1984.

Bowness P, Hawley IC, Morris T, et al: Complete heart block and severe aortic incompetence in relapsing polychondritis. *Arthritis Rheum* 34:97–100, 1991.

Buckley LM, Ades PA: Progressive aortic valve inflammation occurring despite apparent remission of relapsing polychondritis. *Arthritis Rheum* 35:812–814, 1992.

Chang-Miller A, Okamura M, Torres VE, et al: Renal involvement in relapsing polychondritis. *Medicine* 66:202–217, 1987.

Cipriano PR, Alonso DR, Baltaxe HA, et al: Multiple aortic aneurysms in relapsing polychondritis. *Am J Med* 37:1097–1102, 1976.

Dalal BI, Wallace AC, Slinger RP: IgA nephropathy in relapsing polychondritis. *Pathology* 20:85–89, 1988.

Cody DT, Sones DA: Relapsing polychondritis: Audiovestibular manifestations. *Laryngoscope* 81:1208–1222, 1971.

Damiani JM, Levine HL: Relapsing polychondritis-Report of ten cases. Laryngoscope 89:929–941, 1979.

Dolan DL, Lemmon GB Jr, Teitelbaum SL: Relapsing polychondritis: Analytical literature review and studies on pathogenesis. *Am J Med* 41:285–299, 1966.

Ebringer R, Rook G, Swana GT, et al: Autoantibodies to cartilage and type II collagen in relapsing polychondritis and other rheumatic diseases. *Ann Rheum Dis* 40:473–479, 1981.

Esdaile J, Hawkins D, Gold P, et al: Vascular involvement in relapsing polychondritis. *Can Med Assoc J* 116:1019–1022, 1977.

Gardner DG: *Pathological Basis of the Connective Tissue Diseases.* Philadelphia, Lea & Febiger, 1992: 711–715.

Giroux L, Paquin F, Guerard-Desjardins MJ, Lefaivre A: Relapsing polychondritis: An autoimmune disease. *Semin Arthritis Rheum* 13:182–187, 1983.

Grishman E, Churg J, Needle MA, Venkataseshan VS (eds): *The Kidney in Collagen-Vascular Diseases.* New York, Raven Press 1993:189–195.

Herman JH, Dennis MV: Immunopathologic studies in relapsing polychondritis. *J Clin Invest* 52:549–558, 1973.

Isaac BL, Liesegang TJ, Michet CJ Jr: Ocular and systemic findings in relapsing polychondritis. *Ophthalmology* 93:681–689, 1986.

Jaksch-Wartenhorst F: Polychondropathia. *Wien Arch fur Int Med* 6:93–100, 1923.

Kaye RL, Sones DA: Relapsing polychondritis: Clinical and pathologic features of 14 cases. *Ann Intern Med* 60:653–664, 1964.

Lang B, Rothenfusser A, Lanchbury JS, et al: Susceptibility to relapsing polychondritis is associated with HLA-DR4. *Arthritis Rheum* 36:660–664, 1993.

Manna R, Annese V, Ghirlanda G, et al: Relapsing polychondritis with severe aortic insufficiency. *Clin Rheumatol* 4:474–480, 1985.

Marshall DAS, Jackson R, Rae AP, Capell HA: Early aortic valve cusp rupture in relapsing polychondritis. *Ann Rheum Dis* 51:413–415, 1992.

McAdam LP, O'Hanlan MA, Bluestone R, Pearson CM: Relapsing polychondritis: Prospective study of 23 patients and a review of the literature. *Medicine* 55: 193–215, 1976.

Michet CJ Jr: Vasculitis in relapsing polychondritis. *Rheum Dis Clin North Am* 16:441–444, 1990.

Michet CJ Jr, McKenna CH, Luthra HS, O'Fallon WM: Relapsing polychondritis: Survival and predictive role of early disease manifestations. *Ann Intern Med* 104: 74–78, 1986.

Pearson CM, Kline HM, Newcomer VD: Relapsing polychondritis. *N Engl J Med* 263:51–58, 1960.

Riccieri V, Spadaro A, Taccari E, et al: A case of relapsing polychondritis: Pathogenetic considerations. *Clin Exp Rheumatol* 6:95–96, 1988.

Strobel E-S, Lang B, Schumacher M, Peter HH: Cerebral aneurysm in relapsing polychondritis. *J Rheumatol* 19:1482–1483, 1992.

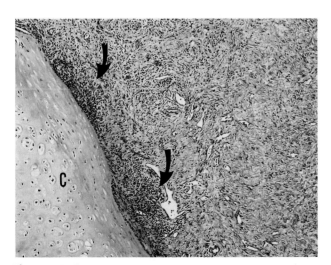

Figure 8.1. Apparently intact cartilage (C) with a predominantly lymphomononuclear cell infiltrate (*arrows*) at the fibrocartilaginous junction of the ear in relapsing polychondritis.

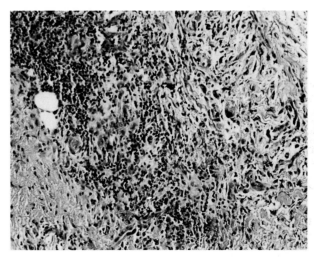

Figure 8.2. Close-up view of the inflammatory infiltrate in relapsing polychondritis.

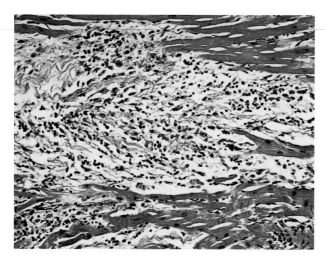

Figure 8.3. Lymphoplasmacytic myocarditis in relapsing polychondritis with heart block.

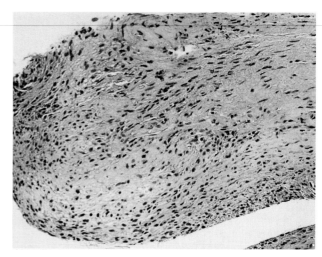

Figure 8.4. Aseptic valvulitis of aortic insufficiency in relapsing polychondritis.

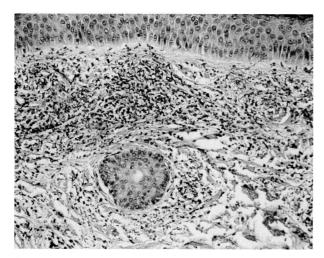

Figure 8.5. Cutaneous leukocytoclastic vasculitis in relapsing polychondritis.

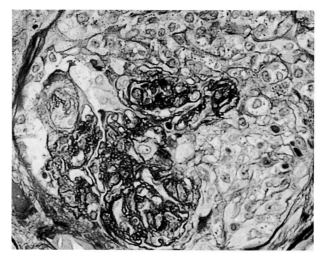

Figure 8.6. Focal segmental necrotizing glomerulonephritis with crescents in relapsing polychondritis. (*Courtesy of Dr. Jacob Churg*)

9. The Vasculitides

DEFINITION AND DIAGNOSIS OF VASCULITIS

Vasculitis has a deceptively simple definition—*inflammation with demonstrable structural injury and, often, occlusive changes of the blood vessels*—but its clinical manifestations can be diverse, complex, and unpredictable. Vasculitis may be generalized ("systemic") or localized ("isolated"). It may occur *de novo* as an essential disorder of the blood vessels (*idiopathic* or *primary* vasculitis) or it may occur in association with a variety of different underlying diseases (*secondary* vasculitis). Thus, the clinical spectrum of vasculitides comprises some of the most interesting and perplexing group of diseases. In the absence of pathognomonic clinical features and laboratory tests, the diagnosis of vasculitis relies heavily on the correct interpretation of the histopathologic changes (biopsies) but these too may not be specific in any given biopsy.

NOSOLOGY AND CLASSIFICATION OF VASCULITIS

Vasculitis is a disease of antiquity. Syphilitic aneurysm was probably first described by the Montpellier professor Antoine Saporta in 1554 when syphilis swept over Europe in the 16th century, and syphilitic aortitis was mentioned in Joseph Hodgson's *Treatise on Diseases of Arteries and Veins* published in London in 1815, antedating the description of arteriosclerosis by Jean-Fédéric Lobstein in 1833.

The prototype of systemic vasculitis, "periarteritis nodosa," was first described in 1866 by Adolf Kussmaul (a clinician) and Rudolf Maier (a pathologist) of Freiburg im Breigau. There was a third person involved in this historic event who should also be remembered, Kussmaul and Maier's patient, a young laborer by the name of Landolin Faist. Feeling grateful for being well treated at the hospital, Faist readily consented to the biopsy of a subcutaneous nodule, which was then a potentially risky procedure in the preantiseptic days. As it happened, the wound on his left leg took nearly three months to heal. In 1903, Ferrari first introduced the now more widely used name "polyarteritis nodosa" to emphasize both the multiplicity of vessel involvement and that the arterial inflammation was often transmural than merely in the outer wall, as the term "periarteritis" might have implied. Involvement of the pulmonary arteries in polyarteritis nodosa was subsequently described by Mönckeberg in 1905, and by Ophüls in 1923, the latter also described involvement of the veins. Dickson, in 1908, first introduced the entity of polyarteritis nodosa to the English-language literature; he also elaborated on the semantic and morphologic differences between "periarteritis" and "polyarteritis."

The descriptions of several other types of systemic vasculitis that followed may be linked to polyarteritis nodosa which is, as it were, the surrogate single parent of the pedigree (Fig. 9.1). Zeek made the first attempt of classification of vasculitis in 1952 by proposing the generic term "necrotizing angiitis" to include, in addition to periarteritis nodosa, *vasculitis of rheumatic disease,* first described by von Glahn and Pappenheimer in 1926; *temporal* (giant cell) *arteritis,* by Horton et al. in 1932; *hypersensitivity vasculitis,* by Rich in 1943; and *allergic granulomatosis and angiitis* by Churg and Strauss in 1951. However, new entities of vasculitis continue to grow in number, creating chaos in terminology, while the etiology and pathogenesis of almost all vasculitides remain unknown or poorly understood and, to date, a classification of vasculitis with universal acceptance is yet to be formulated. Table 9.1 is a practical classification of primary and secondary vasculitis incorporating the predominant type and size of the blood vessel involvement that offers guidelines for when to suspect, how to select the biopsy site, and what to expect in the histopathologic diagnosis of vasculitis.

BIOPSY DIAGNOSIS OF VASCULITIS

The interpretation of histopathologic features of vasculitis in a biopsy is subject to such variables as the examining pathologist's interest and experience, biopsy tissue selection and sample size, chronologic age of the disease process from onset to the time of biopsy and whether or not any drug treatment has begun prior to the biopsy and, ultimately, the histopathologic specificity and variability of any of the major vasculitic syndromes, including the overlapping nature of different vessel size involvement (Fig. 9.2) and their morphologic characteristics (Table 9.2).

This chapter reviews the key diagnostic biopsy features of the seven major systemic and pulmonary vasculitides selected by the American College of Rheumatology's Subcommittee on Classification of Vasculitis: polyarteritis nodosa, Churg-Strauss syndrome, Wegener's granulomatosis, hypersensitivity vasculitis, Schönlein-Henoch syndrome (anaphylactoid purpura), giant

Table 9.1 A Practical Classification of Vasculitis*

Primary Vasculitis

Affecting large, medium, and small blood vessels
- Takayasu arteritis
- Giant cell (temporal) arteritis
- Primary angiitis of the central nervous system

Affecting predominantly medium and small blood vessels
- Polyarteritis nodosa
- Churg-Strauss syndrome
- Wegener's granulomatosis

Affecting predominantly small blood vessels
- Microscopic polyarteritis (microscopic polyangiitis) and capillaritis
- Schönlein-Henoch syndrome (anaphylactoid purpura)
- Leukocytoclastic angiitis

Miscellaneous entities
- Buerger's disease (thromboangiitis obliterans)
- Behçet's disease
- Kawasaki disease (mucocutaneous lymphnode syndrome)

Secondary Vasculitis
- Infection related vasculitis
- Serum sickness or drug/chemical hypersensitivity vasculitis
- Vasculitis associated with rheumatic diseases
- Vasculitis associated with other systemic diseases
- Hypocomplementemic urticarial vasculitis
- Cryoglobulinemia associated vasculitis
- Malignancy related vasculitis
- Post-transplant vasculitis

*Modified from Lie JT. *Arthritis Rheum* 1994;37:181–186.

cell (temporal) arteritis, and Takayasu arteritis; to these is added the *primary angiitis of the central nervous system.* The relative frequencies of these vasculitides, as represented by the author's 2,654 referral consultation cases of all vasculitides, are shown in Fig. 9.3; and they are not dissimilar to the distribution fractions of 1,000 clinical cases from the American College of Rheumatology's multicenter study that created the classification criteria for vasculitis (Fig. 9.4).

Polyarteritis Nodosa

The classic polyarteritis nodosa (PAN) is an idiopathic systemic necrotizing vasculitis of small and medium-sized arteries, very rarely veins, and never the large elastic arteries. Individual susceptibility is associated with hepatitis B virus or hepatitis C virus infection in 10 to 30% of the patients. Involvement of arterioles and the microcirculation, such as the renal glomeruli, are traditionally considered a distinct clinical entity, designated as *microscopic polyarteritis* (MPA). Because MPA may be associated with circulating antineutrophil cytoplasmic antibodies (ANCA) and because it occurs in the lungs as microangiitis or capillaritis, resembling Wegener's granulomatosis, it has become fashionable now to refer to MPA as *microscopic polyangiitis.* Similarly, cutaneous polyarteritis nodosa (CPN) should be differentiated from the systemic PAN by its alleged more benign clinical course and, by definition, absence of visceral involvement. The designation of CPN as a distinct and separate entity is still controversial, however, because many patients with CPN have constitutional symptoms such as arthralgia, myalgia, and/or peripheral neuropathy; and some authors even define CPN as vasculitis limited primarily to the skin, muscles, and/or the peripheral nerves.

The histopathologic lesion defining the classic PAN is a necrotizing vasculitis, usually asymmetrically involving the vessel wall, associated with disruption of the internal elastic lamina, with or without fibrinoid necrosis (Fig. 9.5). The histologic hallmark of PAN includes coexistence of active and healed arteritis, and of unaffected and affected segments (Fig. 9.6). The telltale microaneurysms as the angiographic hallmark of PAN (Fig. 9.7) are more likely found in autopsy or large-organ surgical specimens than in the small muscle, nerve, or rectal mucosal biopsies. Fibrinoid necrosis alone is not specific for PAN; it may be seen in secondary necrotizing vasculitis (as in rheumatoid arthritis or systemic lupus erythematosus) as well in severe forms of systemic or plexogenic pulmonary hypertension.

The biopsy diagnosis of PAN is subject to a number of pitfalls: (1) PAN is characteristically a focal segmental vascular disease and, therefore, small biopsies with negative findings are not uncommon and they do not exclude the disease; (2) histopathologically identical lesions occur in several systemic diseases, notably rheumatoid arthritis and systemic lupus erythematosus; (3) an isolated or localized PAN-type vasculitis, probably due to an Arthus phenomenon, may be found incidentally in such organs as the appendix, gallbladder, or female genital tract; (4) PAN lesions may overlap with other types of primary systemic vasculitis, such as Wegener's granulomatosis and Churg-Strauss syndrome; and (5) certain nonvasculitic conditions, such as fibromuscular dysplasia, atheroembolism, and cardiac myxoma emboli may mimic PAN both clinically and angiographically, biassing the pathologist's over-interpretation of nondiagnostic biopsies.

Contrary to popular belief, the predominant cells of the inflammatory infiltrate in PAN are not granulocytes but macrophages and CD4-positive T-lymphocytes (Fig. 9.8A). The presence of granulocytes is highly variable, ranging from 0 to 40–45% of inflammatory cells, being more plentiful in lesions with fibrinoid necrosis. To further confuse the unwary, PAN, the prototype of necrotizing vasculitis, may occasionally appear as a granulomatous vasculitis (Fig. 9.8B). It is a misconception that MPA manifests only as necrotizing glomerulonephritis and that classic PAN does not involve arterioles (Fig. 9.9). Another misconception is that PAN does not affect the lung; pulmonary PAN occurs in 5 to 10% of cases where the lung has been examined, and it may involve both the bronchial and small pulmonary arteries (Fig. 9.10).

Churg-Strauss Syndrome

Originally described as *allergic granulomatosis and angiitis* in 1951, Churg-Strauss syndrome is a variant of PAN. Drs. Jacob Churg and Lotte Strauss at New York's Mount Sinai Hospital, in the late 1940s, identified a group of autopsy patients diagnosed as PAN who also had asthma or a history of allergy and elevated blood eosinophil counts during life. The characteristic lesions in this group of patients consisted of pulmonary (Fig. 9.11) and systemic (Fig. 9.12) eosinophilic vasculitis and extravascular granulomas, which set them apart from the classic PAN.

We now know that in Churg-Strauss syndrome, while the vasculitis is a constant finding, the extravascular granulomas are found in fewer than 50% of cases; the characteristic lesions may be widespread (systemic form) or isolated (limited form); the subcutaneous and/or cutaneous necrobiotic nodules, sometimes described as "Churg-Strauss granulomas," are quite nonspecific and have been observed more often in a variety of other systemic diseases. Finally, the concept of an overlap syndrome of Wegener's granulomatosis and Churg-Strauss syndrome has been conceived with the false notion that eosinophils are not found in the inflammatory infiltrates of Wegener's granulomatosis. The distinction between Churg-Strauss syndrome and Wegener's granulomatosis is clinically important because the former is more responsive to treatment with corticosteroids alone and has a relatively better prognosis.

Wegener's Granulomatosis

Although the classic Wegener's granulomatosis is characterized by the triad of vasculitis and necrotizing granulomas of the upper and lower respiratory tract, and focal segmental necrotizing glomerulonephritis, virtually any organ in the body may be involved, and the triad may be found concurrently in fewer than 50% of the patients. A "limited" form with lung involvement only at onset is probably a protracted variety of the same disease, because progression to the classic form may eventually occur.

Wegener's granulomatosis is first and foremost a necrotizing inflammatory disease which is often but not invariably granulomatous in character. Vasculitis is a secondary component and occurs in probably less than 50% of the patients, especially in extrapulmonary locations; and it may be granulomatous or nongranulomatous. The biopsy findings of Wegener's granulomatosis vary greatly in different target organs and, also, depending on the sample size of the biopsy. The one truly classic histopathology of Wegener's granulomatosis, a confluent or serpiginous geographic pattern tissue necrosis and vasculitis occurs most consistently in the lung and can only be seen in an open lung biopsy (Fig. 9.13). Focal necrotizing lesions ("microabscesses"), with or without granulomatous inflammation and vasculitis, are found with similar frequencies in pulmonary and extrapulmonary biopsies (Fig. 9.14). A variable number of eosinophils may be present in the inflammatory infiltrate but almost never as prominent as they usually appear in Churg-Strauss syndrome.

Large-vessel thrombosis (Fig. 9.15A) has seldom been emphasized in the literature, but it contributes to regional lung necrosis, infarction, and cavitation; the latter becomes the chest roentgenographic hallmark of Wegener's granulomatosis that is so well known to the clinicians. Microangiitis, or capillaritis (Fig. 9.15B), the cause of diffuse alveolar hemorrhage and at times fulminant lung hemorrhage in Wegener's granulomatosis, was first described in 1960s and has only just received greater attention in recent years. Pulmonary hemorrhage has been estimated to occur in up to one-third of patients; it may be the initial manifestation and the only abnormal lung biopsy finding of Wegener's granulomatosis.

The development of laboratory tests for ANCA in the 1980s has greatly facilitated making a presumptive clinical diagnosis and monitoring disease activity of

Table 9.2. Comparison of the Pathologic Characteristics of Selected Vasculitis Syndromes*

	Polyarteritis Nodosa	Churg-Strauss Syndrome	Wegener's Granulomatosis
Type of vessels involved	Medium and small muscular arteries, and sometimes arterioles	Small arteries and veins, often arterioles and venules	Usually small arteries and veins, sometimes larger vessels
Distribution and localization	Visceral, cutaneous, and, infrequently, cerebral vessels and lung	Upper and lower respiratory tract, viscera, heart, and skin	Upper and lower respiratory tract, often kidney, and infrequently skin, heart, viscera, and brain
Type of vasculitis and inflammatory cell infiltrate	Necrotizing, with mixed cells and few eosinophils, rarely granulomatous	Necrotizing or granulomatous, with mixed cells and prominent eosinophils	Necrotizing or granulomatous, with mixed cells and occasional eosinophils
Special features	Focal segmental involvement of vessels; coexisting acute and healed vascular lesions, or normal and affected vessels; microaneurysms	Extravascular necrotizing granulomas with prominent eosinophils; may manifest as "limited form"	Geographic pattern of tissue necrosis and positive antineutrophil cytoplasmic antibodies; may manifest as "limited form"
Demographic and environmental predisposition	Vascular lesion of infantile polyarteritis is indistinguishable from fatal cases of Kawasaki disease	Most patients have asthma or history of allergy	Occurs in all ages, with a slight male preponderance; associated with HLA-DR2; may respond to antimicrobial agents

*Reproduced with permission from Lie JT. *Arthritis Rheum* 33:1074–1087, 1990.

Wegener's granulomatosis, but it has not obviated the need for biopsy. For biopsy confirmation of the diagnosis of Wegener's granulomatosis, the patient's condition permitting, an open lung biopsy is decidedly preferable to transbronchial biopsy. In head and neck biopsies, which are probably more readily performed than lung biopsies, the Armed Forces Institute of Pathology's experience of 126 biopsies from 70 patients showed that the highest yield was obtained from biopsies of paranasal sinuses (55%), followed by the nasal mucosa (20%) and larynx (18%). However, nonspecific acute and chronic inflammation was the commonest finding (40 to 66%, depending on the biopsy site); vasculitis, tissue necrosis, and granulomatous inflammation were found overall in 26%, 33%, and 42%, respectively, of all head and neck biopsies; combined vasculitis and necrosis in 23%; combined vasculitis and granulomatous inflammation in 21%; and the triad of vasculitis, necrosis, and granulomatous inflammation in only 16% of all head and neck biopsies. Our own experience with head and neck

Hypersensitivity Vasculitis	Henoch-Schönlein Purpura	Giant Cell (Temporal) Arteritis	Takayasu Arteritis
Arterioles and venules, often small arteries and veins	Arterioles and venules, often small arteries and veins	Vessels of all sizes	Elastic arteries and selected muscular arteries
Predominantly skin and less commonly viscera, heart, and synovium	Predominantly skin gastrointestinal, kidney, and synovium	Predominantly temporal arteries, and less often any other large, medium, and small vessels	Aorta, arch vessels, and other major branches (coronary, renal, visceral), and pulmonary arteries
Leukocytoclastic or lymphocytic, with variable number of eosinophils, occasionally granulomatous	Leukocytoclastic, mixed-cell, or lymphocytic, with variable number of eosinophils	Granulomatous, with variable number of giant cells, sometimes only lymphoplasmacytic	Granulomatous, with few giant cells in active phase, and sclerosing fibrosis in chronic stage, with scanty infiltrate
May be associated with myocarditis, interstitial nephritis, or hepatitis	IgA immune deposits in affected tissue	Affected extracranial large vessels indistinguishable from Takayasu arteritis; may form aneurysm or cause dissection	Aneurysmal in 20%; may be segmental, and cause rupture or dissection
Patients may have history of drug or chemical allergy vaccination, or occult malignancy	Predominantly children and young adults	Virtually all patients with temporal arteritis are over age 50; may be clinically asymptomatic	Most commonly in women of childbearing age; more prevalent in the Orient; an important cause of hypertension in adolescents

and orbital biopsies in Wegener's granulomatosis was similar.

Hypersensitivity Vasculitis

Gruber, in 1925, first suggested that hypersensitivity might be involved in the production of vascular lesions in periarteritis nodosa, and the concept received support from experimental studies of sensitization to foreign proteins by Rich and Gregory, in 1943. Zeek, in 1952, was the first to differentiate small-vessel vasculitis of hyper-

sensitivity reaction from periarteritis nodosa in her classification of necrotizing angiitis. The term hypersensitivity vasculitis (HSV) subsequently became synonymous with *small-vessel vasculitis, allergic vasculitis, cutaneous vasculitis,* and *leukocytoclastic vasculitis.* Zeek originally created the term HSV to refer to vasculitis of arterioles and venules developed putatively as an allergic response to a precipitating antigen, such as foreign proteins, drugs, vaccines, and chemicals, others have used the same term to refer to conditions in which cutaneous vasculitis predominates and systemic involvement is absent, undetected, or limited to one or two locations such as the muscle and peripheral nerve.

The histopathology of HSV lacks specificity, as does its etiology. HSV in biopsies may have a predominantly neutrophilic or lymphocytic infiltrate (Fig. 9.16); the former is more often associated with hypocomplementemia than the latter. It is entirely possible that a lymphocytic vasculitis may represent the resolving phase of an immune mechanism mediated neutrophilic vasculitis, as in urticarial vasculitis. Sequential biopsy studies of cutaneous vasculitis have demonstrated that the character of the infiltrate reflects a dynamic process of vascular injury; it can transform from a neutrophilic predominant to lymphocytic predominant cell type in just a few days. Just to muddy the water further, a drug-induced systemic HSV with a granulomatous inflammatory infiltrate also has been observed (Fig. 9.17).

While the term HSV has been used for both cutaneous and visceral small-vessel vasculitis, *leukocytoclastic vasculitis* traditionally applies to a cutaneous vasculitis involving the arterioles and venules, which is characterized by extensive karyorrhexis of the neutrophilic infiltrate with extravasation of erythrocytes and a variable amount of fibrinoid deposits (Fig. 9.18).

Schönlein-Henoch Syndrome (Anaphylactoid Purpura)

The common practice of referring to this disorder as Henoch-Schönlein syndrome (or purpura) is historically incorrect because the description by Johann Lukas Schönlein (1793–1864) of this disease in 1837 antedated that by Eduard Heinrich Henoch (1820–1910) in 1874 by 37 years.

Schönlein-Henoch syndrome (SHS), although it can occur in adults, is essentially a disease of childhood and the most common form of systemic vasculitis in children. It often is preceded by an upper respiratory infection, and it is more common in winter. The syndrome is characterized by nonthrombocytopenic palpable purpura on pressure-bearing areas of the body, cutaneous leukocytoclastic vasculitis, arthritis or arthralgia, gastrointestinal vasculitis, and necrotizing crescenteric glomerulonephritis (Fig. 9.19). The vasculitis is indistinguishable from PAN of the comparable sized blood vessels except that IgA is readily demonstrable by immunofluorescence microscopy in skin and kidney biopsies of patients with SHS. Circulating IgA-containing immune complexes, cryoglobulin, and an IgA ANCA have been demonstrated in some patients. Renal biopsy is impor-

tant as a predictor of end-stage kidney disease in 5 to 10% of the patients.

Giant Cell (Temporal) Arteritis

For reasons not completely understood, giant cell arteritis (GCA) most commonly involves the superficial temporal artery and, hence, the synonyms *temporal arteritis* or *cranial arteritis.* The cause of GCA is unknown. A cellular immune mediated host response has been implicated but not proven. The high prevalence of HLA-DR4 antigen among GCA patients suggests a possible genetic predisposition of the disease. The clinical syndrome of temporal arteritis (or Horton's disease, a term still popular in Europe) and the closely related syndrome of polymyalgia rheumatica (PMR) occur almost invariably in persons over the age of 50 years; both syndromes are two to three times more common in women. Positive temporal artery biopsy for GCA in PMR has been documented in about 30% of North American patients, and in about 60% of Scandinavian and Icelandic patients.

A positive temporal artery biopsy is obligatory to confirm the diagnosis of GCA; and the biopsy may be positive despite the absence of subjective symptoms of temporal arteritis. The biopsy is important not only for establishing a diagnostic baseline but also for assessing disease activity and regulating the drug treatment. Arteritis other than GCA may also be diagnosed serendipitously in temporal artery biopsies intended for the diagnosis of GCA.

The histopathology of GCA has been reviewed periodically in the literature after its initial description more than 60 years ago, but there is still confusion as to what constitutes a positive biopsy for GCA and how to distinguish a healed arteritis from aging change or arteriosclerosis-atherosclerosis of the temporal arteries. The correct interpretation of a temporal artery biopsy requires the observance of the following "Eleven Commandments:"

1. The affected temporal artery, when identified, should be biopsied. Clinical evidence of an affected temporal artery includes tenderness and redness of the overlying skin, cord-like thickening of the artery with or without loss of or diminished pulse. The branch anterior to the main trunk of the selected superficial temporal artery is biopsied with excision of a minimum 2 to 3 cm segment. In the absence of localizing signs and symptoms, the superficial temporal artery on either side may be considered for biopsy.

2. Temporal arteritis may be a bilateral or unilateral disease; involvement of a given artery is characteristically focal and segmental, alternating with skip areas that may be as close together as only 300–350 μm apart; a negative single-sided and short-segment biopsy specimen, therefore, cannot prove the absence of GCA.

3. The excised arterial segment should be straightened out and aligned correctly, untwisted, before placing it into the fixative. After fixation, the artery is cut at right angle to its long axis into 3 mm serial cross-sectional segments, and all segments should be embedded and cut at 5 μm thickness. In bilateral biopsies, the arteries from different sides should be embedded separately and identified. Each glass slide should contain at least three or four "ribbons" of the cut sections from each paraffin block, and at least three or four hematoxylin-eosin stain and one elastic stain glass slides should be routinely processed for an adequate evaluation of the biopsy.

4. The frozen-section technique cannot be relied upon for making a definitive diagnosis, but it may be used as a screening procedure to determine the need for bilateral biopsies.

5. The evidence for a true inflammatory disease of the artery, and not the presence/absence or number of giant cells, is usually considered obligatory for the diagnosis of temporal arteritis.

6. The number of giant cells in temporal arteritis may be solitary or scarce, and not always in proximity to the internal elastic lamina (Fig. 9.20). The giant cells may be plentiful, and some can be readily identified seeming attached to the internal elastic lamina, with or without evidence of phagocytosis of broken fragments of the elastin (Fig. 9.21).

7. About 40 to 45% of positive biopsies for temporal arteritis may show a predominantly lymphocytic infiltrate without evidence of a granulomatous inflammation or giant cells (Fig. 9.22). A GCA (temporal arteritis) sans giant cells has the same clinical significance as a GCA with giant cells. The likelihood of finding giant cells in a positive biopsy is an open-ended search; by cutting through the paraffin blocks, about 20% of the initially giant cell-negative GCA may become giant cell-positive.

8. Close to 99% of all temporal arteritis patients are 50 years or older and, therefore, fragmentation and fraying of the internal elastic lamina *per se,* which is a regular feature of all aging arteries, is not indicative of active or healed arteritis. In temporal arteritis, fragmentation and fraying of the internal elastic lamina is more pronounced, usually asymmetric, and almost always accompanied by an inflammatory infiltrate.

9. Healed temporal arteritis is characterized by intimal fibrosis, medial scarring with the telltale eccentric destruction of the internal elastic lamina from previous injury, associated with usually a scanty residual inflammatory cell infiltrate (Fig. 9.23).

10. Prior corticosteroid treatment up to a 2-week duration has no significant masking effect on the temporal arteritis in biopsies. Occasionally, a histopathologically "active" temporal arteritis may persist for several weeks, or a "recrudescence" may occur after as long as 10 years later in a patient who clinically responded to the initial treatment and had remained asymptomatic.

11. The frequency of "false-negative" temporal artery biopsies is determined by the site selection for biopsy, the minimum length of the arterial segment sampled, whether bilateral biopsies are obtained, the efforts invested in processing the biopsies, and the experience and interest of the examining pathologist. Under optimal conditions and with meticulous preparation of the biopsies, as described, false-negative biopsies should occur in no more than 5% of cases.

Takayasu Arteritis

Takayasu arteritis has many synonyms, including pulseless disease, aortic arch or the middle aorta syndrome, primary aortitis, nonspecific or idiopathic aortitis and aortoarteritis. It is essentially a large-vessel arteritis of unknown etiology, probably an autoimmune disease, occurring six to nine times more commonly in women of reproductive age than in men, and almost ten times more commonly in the Orient and Southeast Asia, Eastern Europe and Latin America, than in North American, Western European and Nordic countries of the world. Takayasu arteritis has occasionally been known to coexist with some of the connective tissue diseases, notably rheumatoid arthritis and systemic lupus erythematosus in young adults; and also with autoimmune inflammatory bowel disease, Crohn's disease in particular.

HLA-Bw52 antigen is associated with 44% of Japanese patients with Takayasu arteritis.

Takayasu arteritis may affect any segment of the aorta, the aortic arch vessels and the pulmonary arteries (Fig. 9.24). In the aorta, aneurysmal dilatation occurs in up to 30% of the patients, and symptomatic aortic insufficiency may be the initial manifestation of the disease. Obstructive disease of the abdominal aorta with involvement of the renal artery ostia in Takayasu arteritis is the most common cause of renovascular hypertension in adolescents and young adults. Takayasu arteritis affects major arteries of the arms and legs not infrequently, but only rarely the visceral arteries and proximal coronary arteries. Involvement of the coronary arteries has led to coronary artery bypass surgery in young adults. The disease is usually diagnosed clinically with the support of compatible aortography and systemic, pulmonary, or coronary angiographic findings. In the past two decades, more frequent operative interventions for complications of aneurysmal and obstructive disease, biopsy diagnosis or confirmation of Takayasu aortitis and arteritis is possible with tissues obtained at surgery, but it is essential that full-thickness arterial walls or the entire endarterectomy specimens be processed for histological evaluation.

The histopathology of Takayasu arteries varies according to the chronologic age of the disease, except when recrudescence occurs. The active or prepulseless phase Takayasu arteritis, as seen in an endarterectomy specimen or full-thickness biopsy samples obtained at arterial reconstructive surgery, is typically a granulomatous panarteritis with a variable number of giant cells (Figs. 9.25 and 9.26), or a lymphoplasmacytic arteritis without giant cells (Fig. 9.27), often associated with multifocal disruption of the medial musculoelastica of the arterial wall and adventitial fibrosis. When a patient presents with symptomatic aortic insufficiency requiring valve replacement, the excised valve cusps should be examined for evidence of an autoimmune lymphoplasmacytic valvulitis (Fig. 9.28). When the aortic vessels are involved in Takayasu arteritis, it is more likely to be the carotid than the subclavian-axillary arteries, compared with extracranial giant cell (temporal) arteritis. Occlusive intimal proliferation and adventitial fibrosis with scanty or absent cellular inflammatory infiltrate is the hallmark of late stage or pulseless phase of the disease (Fig. 9.29) which, to the unwary, may be confused with the banal arteriosclerosis obliterans, especially in more elderly patients.

Primary Angiitis of the Central Nervous System

The central nervous system (CNS) may be the seat of a wide variety of vasculitis (Table 9.3), all but one of which are associated with a known underlying systemic disease (*secondary* vasculitis); the one exception is primary angiitis of the CNS, previously known as *noninfectious, granulomatous* or *isolated* angiitis of the CNS. Although it is primarily an angiitis of the intracranial blood vessels, involvement of extracranial carotid and vertebral arteries occurs occasionally.

Primary angiitis of the CNS is uncommon and, to date, probably fewer than 200 cases have been docu-

Table 9.3 Angiitis of the Central Nervous System*

Primary
  Angiitis of the central nervous system
Secondary
  Infection related angiitis (bacterial, fungal, mycoplasmal, protozoal, rickettsial, viral)
  Associated with systemic vasculitides or systemic diseases
  ■ Giant cell arteritis (temporal arteritis, Takayasu arteritis)
  ■ Polyarteritis nodosa
  ■ Churg-Strauss syndrome
  ■ Wegener's granulomatosis
  ■ Hypersensitivity vasculitis
  ■ Rheumatic connective tissue diseases
  ■ Behçet's disease
  ■ Cogan syndrome
  ■ Sarcoid angiitis
  ■ Inflammatory bowel disease
  Drug related angiitis
  ■ Allopurinol
  ■ Ephedrine
  ■ Amphetamine
  ■ Cocaine
  ■ Heroin
Vasculitis Mimickers
  Antiphospholipid syndrome
  Fibromuscular dysplasia
  Moyamoya disease
  Vasospasm or transient acute arterial hypertension
  Thrombotic thrombocytopenic purpura
  Cardiac myxoma embolism
  Sickle cell anemia
  Radiation vasculopathy
  Acute meningoencephalitis
  Intravascular lymphomatosis (malignant angioendotheliomatosis)

*Modified from Lie JT. *Curr Opin Rheumatol* 1991;3:36–45.

mented in the literature worldwide. The disease occurs in patients in all age groups (mean age 44; range 3 to 75 years); with a 5:3 or 4:3 male preponderance. Primary angiitis of CNS is a serious disease; the majority of patients (60 to 70%) died within the first year of the diagnosis, and about one-third to one-half of survivors have significant neurological deficits. Most of the cases reported in the literature were diagnosed clinically and angiographically, or at autopsy. The importance of histologic confirmation has been emphasized by many investigators, particularly to eliminate a variety of angiitis mimickers (Table 9.3). Biopsy diagnosis, however, is limited by the inconclusiveness of a negative finding because the CNS angiitis is typically a focal segmental disease and the small sample size of brain biopsies may not capture the lesions.

In a positive brain biopsy, primary angiitis of the CNS affects the small and medium-sized arteries, and only rarely veins and venules, of the brain and meninges. A wide assortment of histologically heterogeneous angiitis maybe seen in the same biopsy, given a large enough sized sample: granulomatous angiitis (Fig. 9.30) and lymphocytic angiitis (Fig. 9.31), lymphocytic and healed angiitis (Fig. 9.32), or granulomatous angiitis and necrotizing angiitis; and both the foreign-body and Langhans giant cells may be found in granulomatous angiitis (Fig. 9.33).

To date, there have been twelve reported cases of primary angiitis of the CNS involving the spinal cord, of which nine were associated with cerebral angiitis and three were not. In the majority of these cases, the spinal cord involvement was clinically overshadowed by overt manifestations of cerebral involvement, and the diagnosis was made unexpectedly when signs and symptoms of myelopathy necessitated a spinal cord biopsy. The spinal cord biopsy may show a granulomatous angiitis with giant cells (Fig. 9.34) and/or a lymphocytic angiitis without giant cells (Fig. 9.35) in the same specimen. Microvascular thromboses (Fig. 9.36) are often observed in positive brain and spinal cord biopsies for primary angiitis of the CNS.

BIBLIOGRAPHY

Achkar AA, Lie JT, Hunder GG, et al: How does previous corticosteroid treatment affect the biopsy findings in giant cell (temporal) arteritis? *Ann Intern Med* 120: 987–992, 1994.

Achkar AA, Lie JT, Gabriel SE, Hunder GG: Giant cell arteritis involving the facial artery. *J Rheumatol* 22: 363–366, 1995.

Ansell BM, Bacon PA, Lie JT, Yazici H (eds): *The Vasculitides: Science and Practice.* London, Chapman & Hall, 1996, 447 pp.

Baldursson O, Steinsson K, Björnsson J, Lie JT: Temporal arteritis in Iceland: An epidemiological and histopathological analysis. *Arthritis Rheum* 37: 1007–1012, 1994.

Cohle SD, Harris LS, Lie JT: Sudden death associated with aortitis and fibrosclerotic disease of the conduction system. *Arch Pathol Lab Med* 116:1163–1166, 1992.

Dunn PM: Dr. Euard Henoch (1820–1910) of Berlin: Pioneer of German paediatrics. *Arch Dis Child* 74: F149–F150, 1996.

Ettlinger RE, Nelson AM, Burke EC, Lie JT: Polyarteritis nodosa in childhood: a clinical pathologic study. *Arthritis Rheum* 22:820–825, 1979.

Gabriel SE, Achkar AA, Lie JT, et al: The use of clinical characteristics to predict the result of temporal artery biopsy among patients with suspected giant cell arteritis. *J Rheumatol* 22:93–96, 1995.

Hall S, Barr W, Lie JT, et al: Takayasu arteritis: a study of 32 North American patients. *Medicine* 64:89–99, 1985.

Hall S, Persellin S, Lie JT, et al: The therapeutic impact of temporal artery biopsy. *Lancet* 2:1217–1220, 1983.

Henoch EH: Über eine eigenthumliche form von purpura. *Berlin klin Wochenschr* 11:641–643, 1874.

Hunder GG, Lie JT: The vasculitides. *Cardiovasc Clin* 13(2):261–291, 1983.

Hunder GG, Lie JT: Systemic vasculitis and related disorders. In Cohen AS, Bennett JC (eds): *Rheumatology and Immunology,* ed 2. Orlando, Grune & Stratton, 1986:279–288.

Hunder GG, Lie JT: The vasculitic syndrome. In Stein JH (ed): *Internal Medicine,* ed 4. St. Louis, Mosby-Year Book, 1994:2430–2441.

Hunder GG, Lie JT, Goronzy J, Weyand C: Pathogenesis of giant cell arteritis. *Arthritis Rheum* 36:757–761, 1993.

Huston KA, Combs JJ, Lie JT, Giuliani ER: Left atrial myxoma simulating peripheral vasculitis. *Mayo Clin Proc* 53:752–756, 1978.

Huston KA, Hunder GG, Lie JT, et al: Temporal arteritis: a 25-year epidemiologic, clinical and pathologic study. *Ann Intern Med* 88:162–167, 1978.

Igarashi T, Nagaoka S, Lie JT, et al: Aortitis syndrome (Takayasu aortitis) associated with systemic lupus erythematosus. *J Rheumatol* 16:1579–1583, 1989.

Inwards DJ, Piepgras DG, Lie JT, et al: Granulomatous angiitis of the spinal cord associated with Hodgkin's disease. *Cancer* 68:1318–1322, 1991.

Kalina PH, Lie JT, Campbell RJ, Garrity JA: The diagnostic value and limitations of orbital biopsy in Wegener's granulomatosis. *Ophthalmology* 99:120–124, 1992.

Kaneishi N, Howell LP, Lie JT, et al: Fine needle aspiration cytology of pulmonary Wegener's granulomatosis with biopsy correlation. *Acta Cytologica* 39:1094–1100, 1995.

Lakhanpal S, Conn DL, Lie JT: Clinical and prognostic significance of vasculitis as an early manifestation of connective tissue disease syndromes. *Ann Intern Med* 101:743–748, 1984.

Lakhanpal S, Lie JT, Karper RE, et al: Priapism as a manifestation of isolated genital vasculitis. *J Rheumatol* 18:902–903, 1991.

Lesser RS, Aledort D, Lie JT: Non-giant cell arteritis of the temporal artery presenting as the polymyalgia rheumatica-temporal arteritis syndrome. *J Rheumatol* 22:2177–2182, 1995.

Lie JT: Nosology of pulmonary vasculitides. *Mayo Clin Proc* 52:520–522, 1977.

Lie JT: Disseminated visceral giant cell arteritis: Histopathologic description and differentiation from other granulomatous vasculitides. *Am J Clin Pathol* 69:299–305, 1978.

Lie JT: The structure of the normal vascular system and its reactive changes. In Juergens JL, Spittell JA Jr, Fairbairn II (eds): Allen-Barker-Hines *Peripheral Vascular Diseases,* ed 5. Philadelphia, W B Saunders, 1980: 237–251.

Lie JT: The classification of vasculitis and a reappraisal of allergic granulomatosis and angiitis (Churg-Strauss syndrome). *Mount Sinai J Med* 53:429–439, 1986.

Lie JT: The classification and diagnosis of vasculitis in large and medium-sized blood vessels. *Pathol Annu* 22 (part 1):125–162, 1987.

Lie JT: Thromboangiitis obliterans (Buerger's disease) in women. *Medicine* 66:65–72, 1987.

Lie JT: Coronary vasculitis: A review in the current scheme of classification of vasculitis. *Arch Pathol Lab Med* 111:224–233, 1987.

Lie JT: Segmental Takayasu (giant cell) aortitis with rupture and limited dissection. *Hum Pathol* 18:1183–1185, 1987.

Lie JT: Thromboangiitis obliterans in an elderly man after cessation of cigarette smoking. *Angiology* 38:864–867, 1987.

Lie JT: Isolated polyarteritis nodosa of testis in hairy cell leukemia. *Arch Pathol Lab Med* 112:646–647, 1988.

Lie JT: Classification and immunodiagnosis of vasculitis: A new solution or promises unfulfilled? *J Rheumatol* 15:728–732, 1988.

Lie JT: Thromboangiitis obliterans (Buerger's disease) revisited. *Pathol Annu* 23 (part 2):257–291, 1988.

Lie JT: Classification of pulmonary angiitis and granulomatosis: Histopathologic perspectives. *Semin Respir Med* 10:111–121, 1989.

Lie JT: Systemic and isolated vasculitis: A rational approach to classification and pathologic diagnosis. *Pathol Annu* 24 (part 1): 25–114, 1989.

Lie JT: The rise and fall and resurgence of thromboangiitis obliterans (Buerger's disease). *Acta Pathol Jpn* 39:153–158, 1989.

Lie JT: Vasculopathy in the antiphospholipid syndromes: Thrombosis or vasculitis, or both? *J Rheumatol* 16:713–715, 1989.

Lie JT: Diagnostic histopathology of major systemic and pulmonary vasculitic syndromes. *Rheum Dis Clin North Am* 16:269–292, 1990.

Lie JT: Illustrated histopathologic classification criteria for selected vasculitic syndromes. *Arthritis Rheum* 33: 1074–1087, 1990.

Lie JT: Angiitis of the central nervous system. *Curr Opin Rheumatol* 3:36–45, 1991.

Lie JT: Vasculitis and the gut: Unwitting partners or strange bedfellows. *J Rheumatol* 18:647–649, 1991.

Lie JT: Takayasu arteritis. In Churg A, Churg J (eds): *Systemic Vasculitides.* New York, Igaku-Shoin, 1991: 159–179.

Lie JT: Infection-related vasculitis. In Churg A, Churg J (eds): *Systemic Vasculitides.* New York, Igaku-Shoin, 1991:243–256.

Lie JT: Vasculitis, 1815 to 1991:Classification and diagnostic specificity (The 1991 Dunlop-Dottridge Lecture) *J Rheumatol* 19:83–89, 1992.

Lie JT: Vasculitis simulators and vasculitis look-alikes. *Curr Opin Rheumatol* 4:47–55, 1992.

Lie JT: Primary (granulomatous) angiitis of the central nervous system: A clinicopathologic analysis of 15 new cases and review of the literature. *Hum Pathol* 23:164–171, 1992.

Lie JT: Vascular involvement in Behçet's disease: Arterial and venous and blood vessels of all sizes. *J Rheumatol* 19:341–343, 1992.

Lie JT: Malignant angioendotheliomatosis (intravascular lymphomatosis) simulating primary angiitis of the central nervous system. *Arthritis Rheum* 35:831–834, 1992.

Lie JT: Retroperitoneal polyarteritis nodosa presenting as ureteral obstruction. *J Rheumatol* 19:1628–1631, 1992.

Lie JT: Giant cell temporal arteritis in a Laotian Chinese. *J Rheumatol* 19:1651–1652, 1992.

Lie JT: Classification criteria and histopathologic specificity of major vasculitic syndromes. In Tanabe T (ed): *Intractable Vasculitis Syndromes* (Proceedings of An International Symposium). Sapporo, Japan, Hokkaido University Press, 1993:17–25.

Lie JT: Limited forms of Churg-Strauss syndrome. *Pathol Annu* 28(part 2):199–220, 1993.

Lie JT: Pulmonary involvement in systemic vasculitis. In Saldana M (ed): *Pathology of Pulmonary Disease.* Philadelphia, J B Lippincott Company, 1994:781–790.

Lie JT: Nomenclature and classification of vasculitis: Plus ça change, plus c'est la même chose. *Arthritis Rheum* 37:181–186, 1994.

Lie JT: When is arteritis of the temporal artery not temporal arteritis? *J Rheumatol* 21:186–189, 1994.

Lie JT: Vasculitis in antiphospholipid syndrome: Culprit or consort? *J Rheumatol* 21:397–399, 1994.

Lie JT: Classification and histopathologic specificity of vasculitis. *Cardiovasc Pathol* 3: 191–196, 1994.

Lie JT: Occidental (temporal) and oriental (Takayasu) giant cell arteritis. *Cardiovasc Pathol* 3:227–240, 1994.

Lie JT: Systemic, pulmonary, and cerebral vasculitis. In Stehbens WE, Lie JT (eds): *Vascular Pathology.* London, Chapman & Hall, 1995:489–516.

Lie JT: Simultaneous clinical manifestations of malignancy and giant cell arteritis in a young woman. *J Rheumatol* 22:367–369, 1995.

Lie JT: Bilateral juvenile temporal arteritis. *J Rheumatol* 22:774–776, 1995.

Lie JT: Aortic and extracranial large-vessel giant cell arteritis: A review of 72 cases with histopathologic documentation. *Semin Arthritis Rheum* 24:422–431, 1995.

Lie JT: Vasculitis look-alikes and pseudovasculitic syndromes. *Curr Diag Pathol* 2:78–85, 1995.

Lie JT: Histopathologic specificity of systemic vasculitis. *Rheum Dis Clin North Am* 21:883–909, 1995.

Lie JT: Isolated necrotizing and granulomatous vasculitis causing ischemic bowel disease in primary Sjögren's syndrome. *J Rheumatol* 22:2375–2376, 1995.

Lie JT: Classification and histopathologic specificity of systemic vasculitis. In Ansell BM, Bacon PA, Lie JT, Yazici H (eds): *The Vasculitides: Science and Practice.* London, Chapman & Hall, 1996:21–36.

Lie JT: Takayasu arteritis: A current update. In Ansell BM, Bacon PA, Lie JT, Yazici H (eds): *The Vasculitides: Science and Practice.* London, Chapman & Hall, 1996:181–198.

Lie JT: Angiitis of the central nervous system. In Ansell BM, Bacon PA, Lie JT, Yazici H (eds): *The Vasculitides; Science and Practice.* London, Chapman & Hall, 1996:246–263.

Lie JT: Vasculitis associated with infectious agents. *Curr Opin Rheumatol* 8:26–29, 1996.

Lie JT; Temporal artery biopsy diagnosis of giant cell arteritis: Lessons from 1109 biopsies. ASCP *Ann Rev Pathol* 1996:69–86.

Lie JT: Isolated pulmonary Takayasu arteritis. *Mod Pathol* 9:469–474, 1996.

Lie JT: Primary cutaneous granulomatous phlebitis: Unmasking of a masked villain. *Mod Pathol* 9:719–724, 1996.

Lie JT, Bayardo RJ: Isolated eosinophilic coronary arteritis and eosinophilic myocarditis: A limited form of Churg-Strauss syndrome. *Arch Pathol Lab Med* 113:199–201, 1989.

Lie JT, Brown AL Jr, Carter ET: Spectrum of aging changes in temporal arteries: Its significance in interpretation of biopsy of temporal artery. *Arch Pathol Lab Med* 90:278–285, 1970.

Lie JT, Churg J: The vasculitides. In Edwards JE, Edwards WD, Lie JT, Titus JL (eds): *Cardiovascular Pathology.* New York , Igaku-Shoin (in press).

Lie JT, Dixit RK: Nonsteroidal antiinflammatory drug (NSAID) induced hypersensitivity vasculitis clinically mimicking temporal arteritis. *J Rheumatol* 23:183–185, 1996.

Lie JT, Failoni DD, Davis DC Jr: Temporal arteritis with giant cell aortitis, coronary arteritis, and myocardial infarction. *Arch Pathol Lab Med* 110:857–860, 1986.

Lie JT, Gordon LP, Titus JL: Juvenile temporal arteritis: A biopsy study of four cases. *JAMA* 234:496–499, 1975.

Lie JT, Kobayashi S, Tokano Y, Hashimoto H: Systemic and cerebral vasculitis coexisting with disseminated coagulopathy in systemic lupus erythematosus associated with antiphospholipid syndrome. *J Rheumatol* 22:2173–2176, 1995.

Lie JT, Nagal S: Eosinophilic temporal arteritis in Churg-Strauss syndrome: A new entity. *J Rheumatol* 21:366–367, 1994.

Lie JT, Tokugawa DA: Bilateral lower limb gangrene and stroke as initial manifestations of systemic giant cell arteritis in an African American. *J Rheumatol* 22:363–366, 1995.

Olin JW, Lie JT: Thromboangiitis obliterans (Buerger's disease). In Loscalzo J, Creager MA, Dzau (eds): *Vascular Medicine,* ed 2. Boston, Little, Brown, and Co, 1996:1033–1049.

Owyang C, Miller LJ, Lie JT, Fleming CR: Takayasu's arteritis in Crohn's disease. *Gastroenterology* 76: 825–828, 1979.

Papaioannou CC, Hunder GG, Lie JT: Vasculitis of the gallbladder in a 70-year-old man with giant cell (temporal) arteritis. *J Rheumatol* 6:71–75, 1979.

Rosenow EC III, Lie JT: The pulmonary vasculitides. In Fishman AP (ed): *Pulmonary Diseases and Disorders.* New York, McGraw-Hill, 1992:465–474.

Rushing L, Schoen FJ, Hirsch A, Lie JT: Granulomatous aortic valvulitis associated with aortic insufficiency in Takayasu aortitis. *Hum Pathol* 22:1050–1053, 1991.

Schönlein JL: *Allgemeine und Specielle Pathologie und Therapie,* vol 2. Freyburg, 1837:48.

Tomlinson FH, Lie JT, Nienhuis B, et al: Juvenile temporal arteritis revisited. *Mayo Clin Proc* 69:445–447, 1994.

Walz-LeBlanc BAE, Keystone EC, Lie JT, et al: Polyarteritis nodosa clinically masquerading as temporal arteritis with lymphadenopathy. *J Rheumatol* 21:949–952, 1994.

Webb J, Lie JT: Giant cell arteritis in the young. *J Rheumatol* 23:197, 1996.

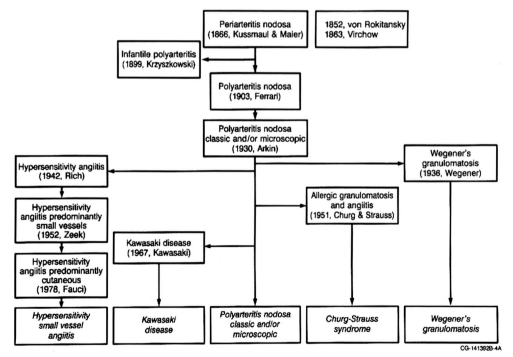

Figure 9.1. A family tree of systemic vasculitis with periarteritis nodosa as the surrogate single parent. (*Reproduced with permission from Lie JT. J Rheumatol* 1991;19:83–89)

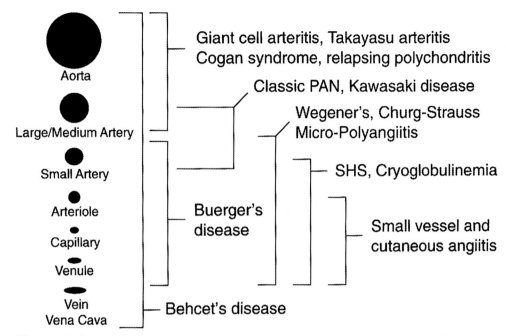

Figure 9.2. Schematic representation of overlapping blood vessel involvement in major systemic vasculitides. (*Redrawn with modification from Mandell BF, Hoffman GS. Rheum Dis Clin North Am* 1994; 20:409–442)

Relative Frequencies of Vasculitis According to ACR Classification

	n	%
Polyarteritis Nodosa	204	7.7
Churg-Strauss Syndrome	116	4.4
Wegener's Granulomatosis	216	8.1
Hypersensitivity Vasculitis	189	7.1
Schönlein-Henoch Syndrome (Anaphylactoid Purpura)	74	2.8
Giant Cell (Temporal) Arteritis	1,109	41.8
Takayasu Arteritis	117	4.4
Kawasaki Disease	54	2.0
Primary Angiitis of the Central Nervous System	32	1.2
Thromboangiitis Obliterans (Buerger's Disease)	178	6.7
Vasculitis of Connective Tissue Diseases and Other Systemic Disorders	365	13.8
TOTAL	2,654	100.0

Figure 9.3. Relative frequencies (number of cases and percents) of vasculitis according to the ACR (American College of Rheumatology) classification in author's 2,654 biopsy-proven referral consultation cases.

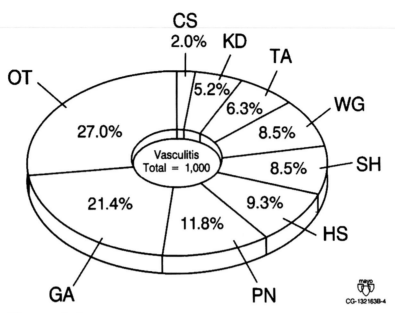

Figure 9.4. Distribution of 1,000 clinical cases of vasculitis according to the ACR (American College of Rheumatology) classification categories. CS: Churg-Strauss syndrome; KD: Kawasaki disease; TA: Takayasu arteritis; WG: Wegener's granulomatosis; SH: Schönlein-Henoch syndrome; HS: hypersensitivity vasculitis; PN: polyarteritis nodosa; GA: giant cell (temporal) arteritis; OT: other vasculitis of unspecified type.

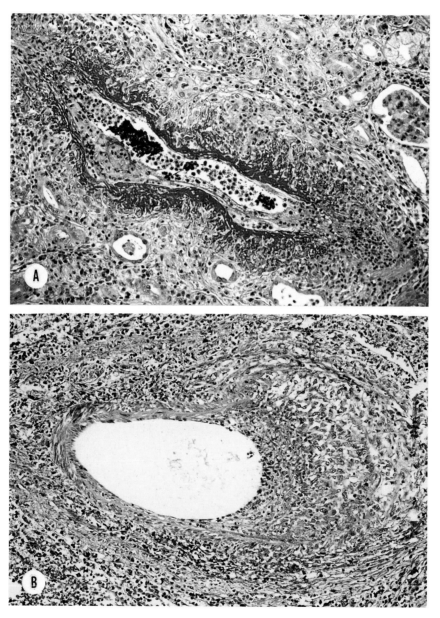

Figure 9.5. Classic polyarteritis nodosa, **(A)** with and **(B)** without overt fibrinoid necrosis.

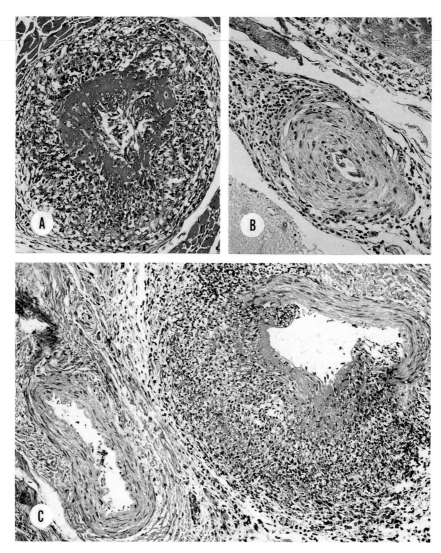

Figure 9.6. Classic polyarteritis nodosa with coexisting **(A)** active and **(B)** healing lesions in different organs; and in **(C)**, affected (*right*) and unaffected (*left*) arteries in the same field.

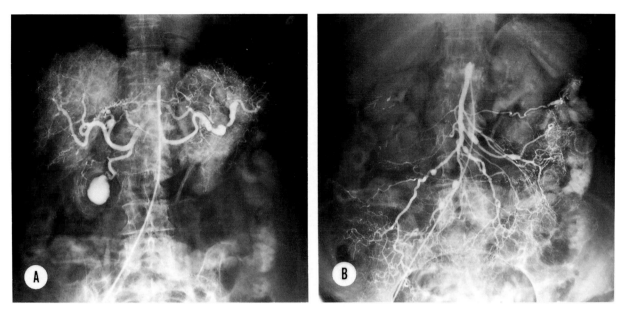

Figure 9.7. Multiple microaneurysms as angiographic hallmark of polyarteritis nodosa in renal (*left*) and superior mesenteric (*right*) arteries and branches of the same patient.

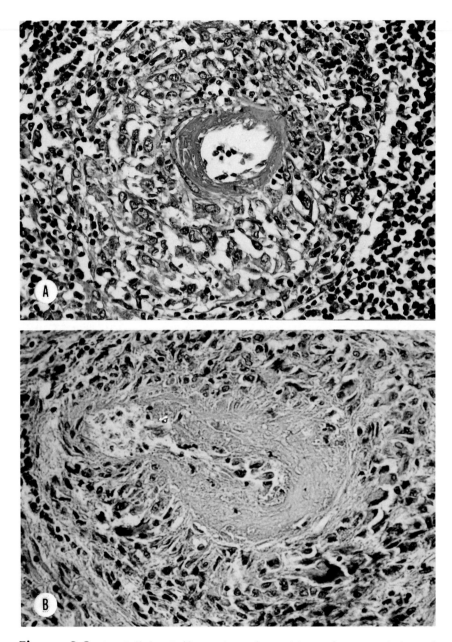

Figure 9.8. A. Cellular infiltrate in polyarteritis nodosa consisting of macrophages and CD4-positive T lymphocytes. **B.** Polyarteritis nodosa with granulomatous infiltrate and giant cell.

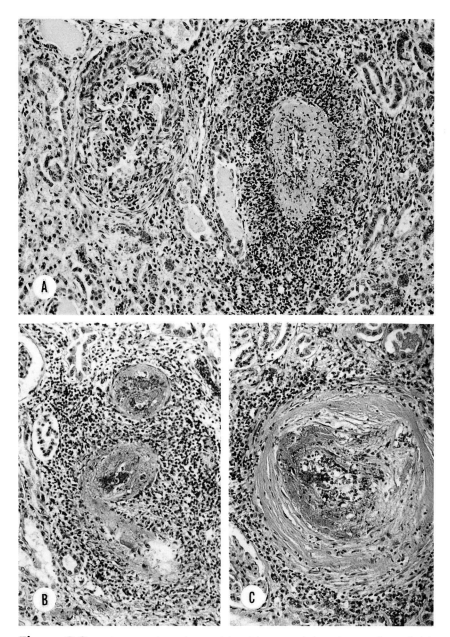

Figure 9.9. Microscopic polyarteritis with necrotizing glomerulonephritis (*left*) and arteriolar lesion (*right*) in the same field **(A).** Classic polyarteritis with involvement of arterioles **(B)** and a small artery **(C)** in the same kidney.

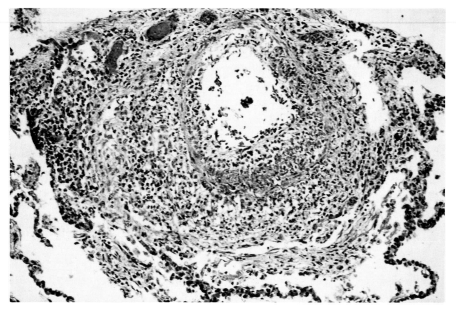

Figure 9.10. Polyarteritis nodosa involving a small pulmonary artery in the lung parenchyma.

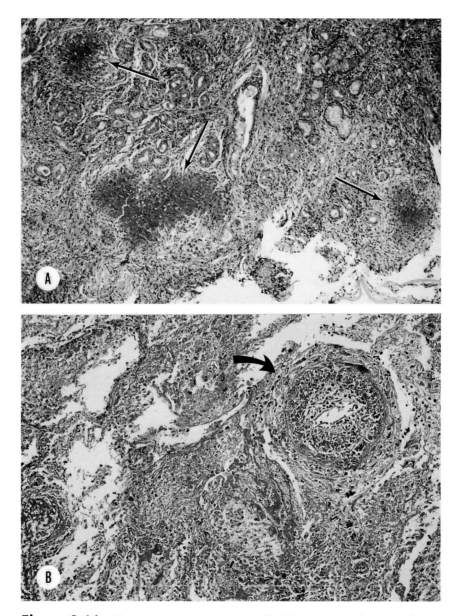

Figure 9.11. Churg-Strauss syndrome with **(A)** extravascular granulomas (*arrows*) and **(B)** granulomatous vasculitis (*arrow*) in an open lung biopsy.

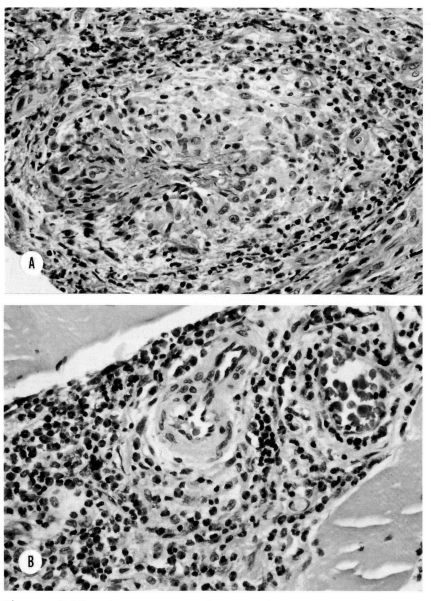

Figure 9.12. Churg-Strauss syndrome with extravascular granuloma (**A**) and eosinophilic vasculitis (**B**) in a muscle biopsy.

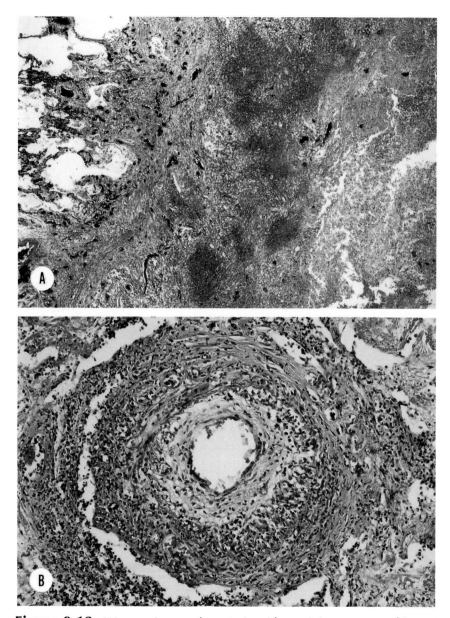

Figure 9.13. Wegener's granulomatosis with serpiginous geographic pattern tissue necrosis (**A**) and granulomatous necrotizing vasculitis (**B**) in an open lung biopsy.

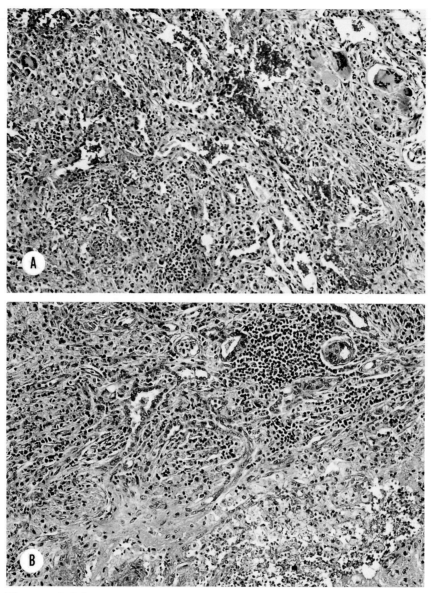

Figure 9.14. Focal necrotizing lesions (microabscesses) in Wegener's granulomatosis, **(A)** with and **(B)** without granulomatous inflammation and giant cells.

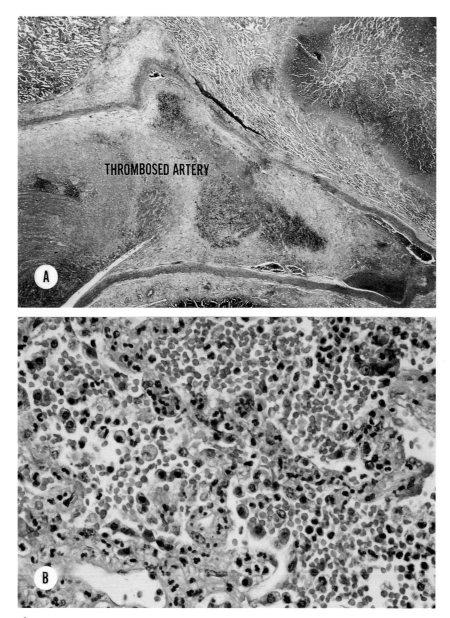

Figure 9.15. Contrasting vascular lesions: **(A)** large-vessel arterial thrombosis and **(B)** capillaritis with alveolar hemorrhage of Wegener's granulomatosis in an open lung biopsy.

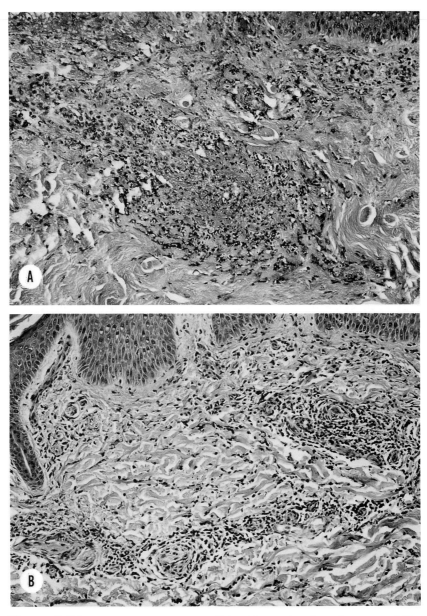

Figure 9.16. Hypersensitivity vasculitis with predominantly neutrophilic (**A**) and lymphocytic (**B**) inflammatory infiltrate.

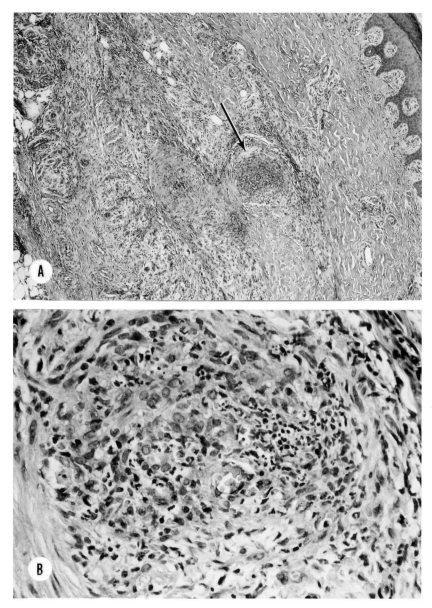

Figure 9.17. A. Phenytoin-induced hypersensitivity vasculitis with a granulomatous infiltrate (*arrow*). **B.** Close-up view of granulomatous cutaneous vasculitis in a skin biopsy.

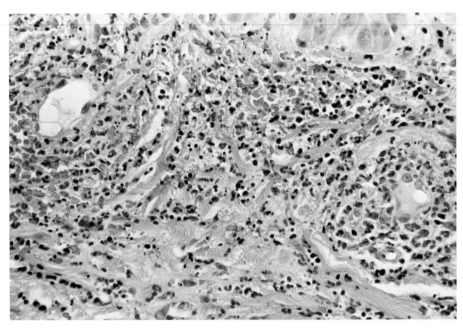

Figure 9.18. Cutaneous leukocytoclastic vasculitis with granulocyte karyorrhexis and erythrocyte extravasation.

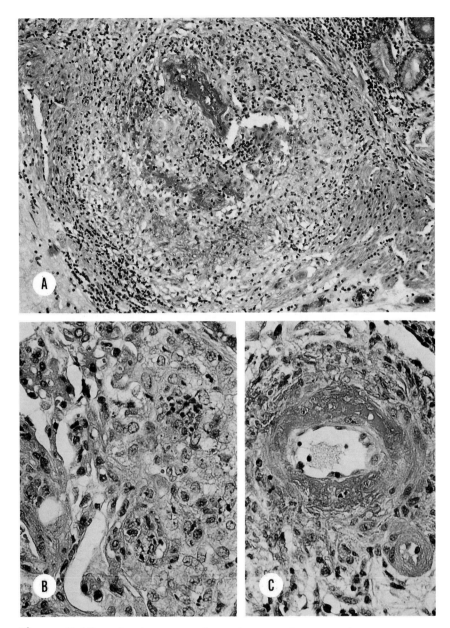

Figure 9.19. Schönlein-Henoch syndrome with intestinal necrotizing vasculitis (**A**), necrotizing glomerulonephritis (**B**), and renal arteriolitis (**C**).

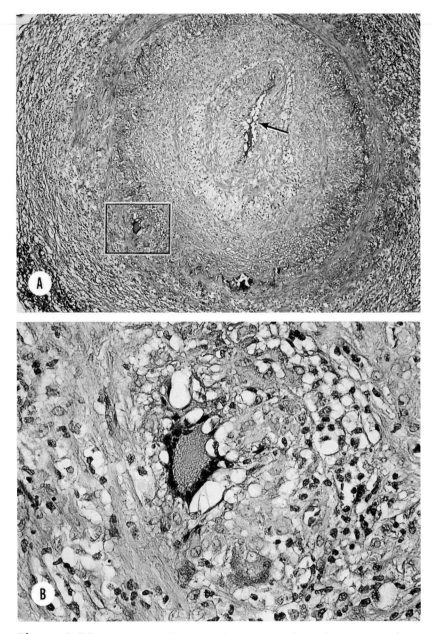

Figure 9.20. **A.** Giant cell temporal arteritis with occlusive intimal proliferation (*arrow*) and granulomatous inflammation in the media. **B.** Close-
up view of the boxed area in **A** to show the granuloma comprising histiocytes and giant cells.

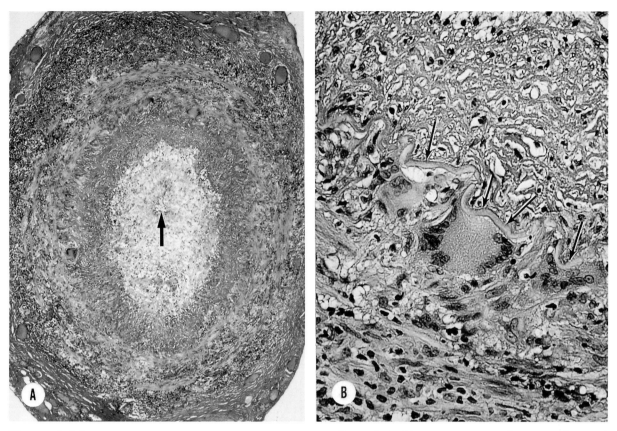

Figure 9.21. **A.** Giant cell temporal arteritis with a virtually occluded lumen (*arrow*) and a circumferential band of fibrinoid necrosis around the intima-media junction. **B.** Close-up view to show attachment of the internal elastic lamina fragment to giant cells (*arrows*).

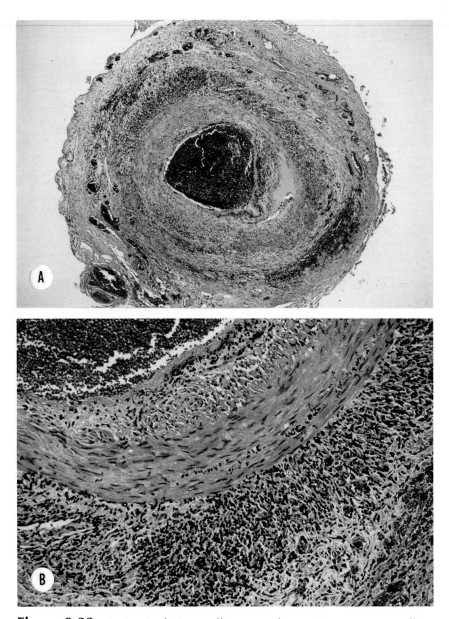

Figure 9.22. A. Atypical giant cell (temporal) arteritis sans giant cells. **B.** Close-up view of a quadrant of the arterial wall with an intense lymphocytic infiltrate but no giant cells.

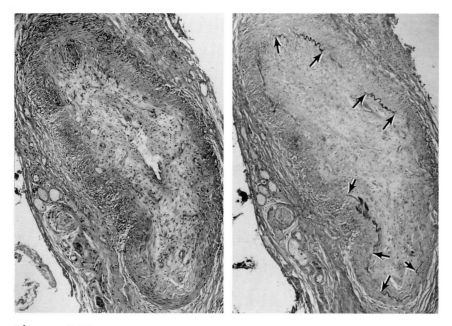

Figure 9.23. Matching hematoxylin-eosin (*left*) and elastic stain (*right*) photomicrographs of a healed giant cell temporal arteritis. Note the vascularized occlusive intimal proliferation in the left panel and asymmetric medial scarring with disruption of the internal elastic lamina (*arrows*) in the right panel.

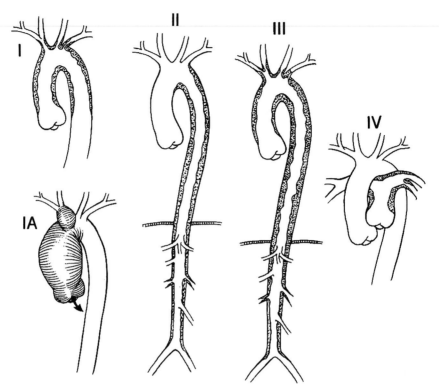

Figure 9.24. Anatomic classification of Takayasu aortitis-arteritis: type I, with involvement of the ascending aorta and aortic arch arterial branches; type IA, variant with aneurysmal ascending aorta; type II, with involvement of the descending thoracic and abdominal aorta; type III, with combined involvement of types I and II; type IV, with involvement of the pulmonary arteries.

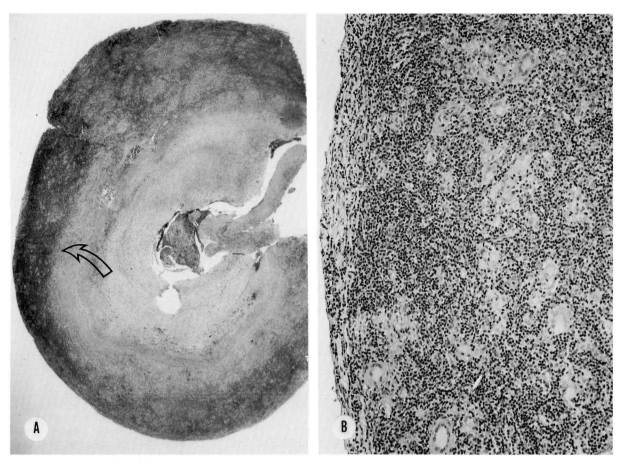

Figure 9.25. **A.** Endarterectomy specimen of Takayasu arteritis with occlusive fibrous intimal proliferation and a granulomatous panarteritis. **B.** Close-up view of the medial granulomatous inflammation with numerous giant cells in the area indicated by arrow in **A.**

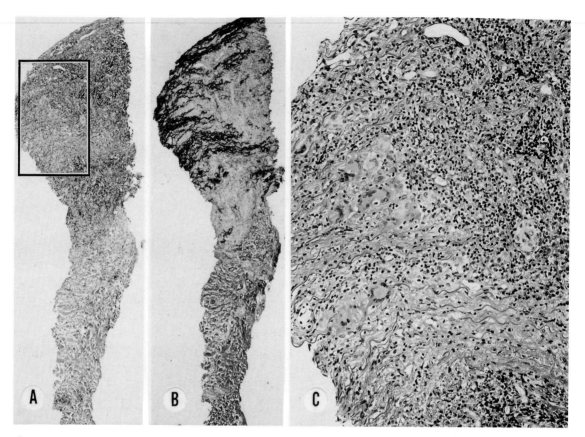

Figure 9.26. Matching hematoxylin-eosin (**A**) and elastic stain (**B**) sections of a full-thickness sliver of biopsy obtained at aortic reconstruction surgery for Takayasu aortitis that show active granulomatous arteritis with patchy disruption of the medial musculoelastic lamellae. **C.** Close-up view of the boxed area in **A** to show the granulomatous inflammation with giant cells.

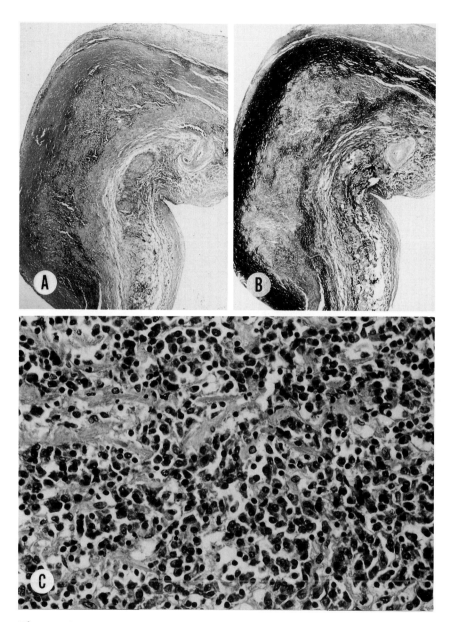

Figure 9.27. Matching hematoxylin-eosin (**A**) and elastic stain (**B**) sections of Takayasu aortitis specimen obtained at valve replacement for aortic insufficiency show a diffuse medial infiltrate in **A** corresponding to a wide band of disruption/effacement of musculoelastic lamellae in **B;** and **C** is close-up view of the medial lymphoplasmacytic infiltrate without giant cells.

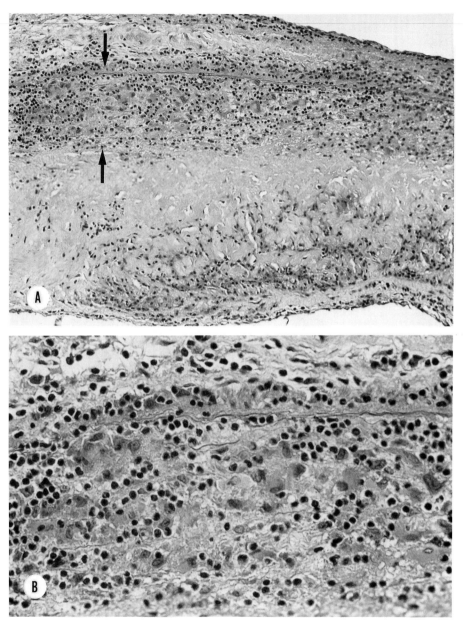

Figure 9.28. A. Granulomatous valvulitis in a specimen obtained at valve replacement for aortic insufficiency in Takayasu aortitis. **B.** Close-up view of giant cells in valvulitis (*arrows* in **A**).

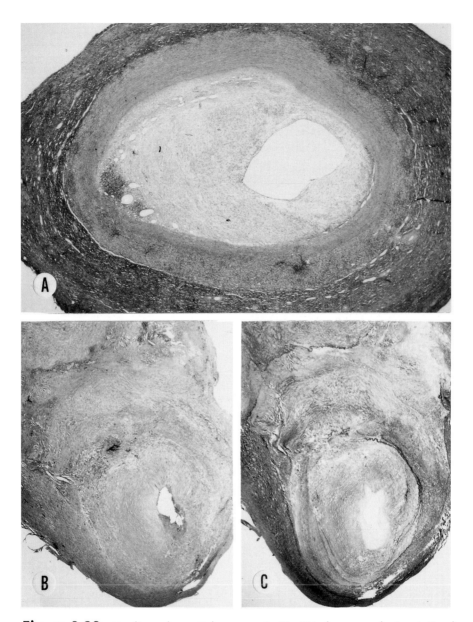

Figure 9.29. Healing phase Takayasu arteritis **(A)** shows occlusive intimal proliferation with scanty residual inflammatory infiltrate and a thick collar of adventitial fibrosis. Hematoxylin-eosin **(B)** and elastic stain **(C)** matching sections of end-stage Takayasu aortitis involving the proximal renal artery show only occlusive fibrosis with absence of inflammatory infiltrate that could be confused with chronic arteriosclerosis obliterans.

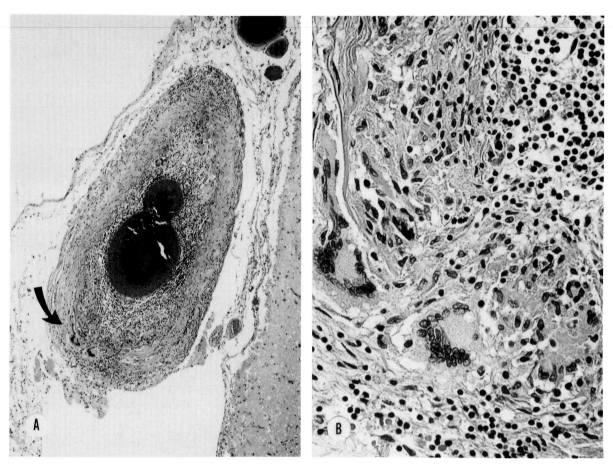

Figure 9.30. **A.** Granulomatous primary angiitis of the CNS. **B.** Close-up view of the area in **A,** indicated by arrow, to show the giant cells in the inflammatory infiltrate.

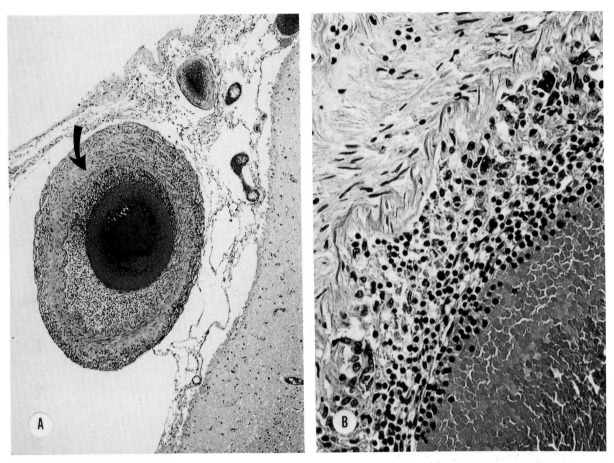

Figure 9.31. **A.** Lymphocytic primary angiitis of the CNS. **B.** Close-up view of the area in **A,** indicated by arrow, to show lymphocytic infiltrate without giant cells.

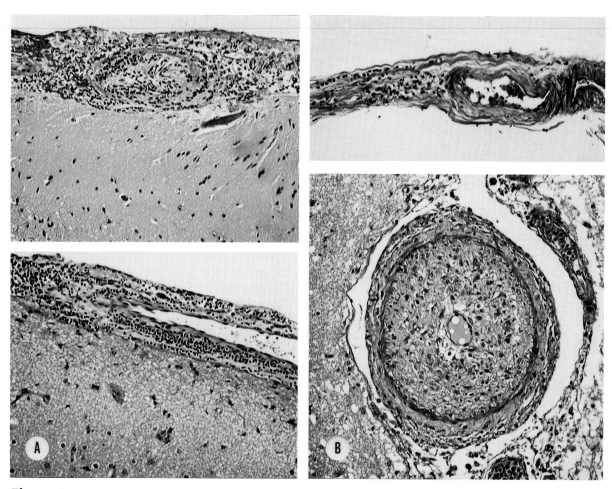

Figure 9.32. Variations of cerebral primary angiitis: **A.** Meningeal lymphocytic angiitis with (*above*) and without (*below*) fibrinoid necrosis. **B.** Meningeal perivascular lymphocytic infiltrate (*above*) and intracerebral healing or healed vasculitis (*below*).

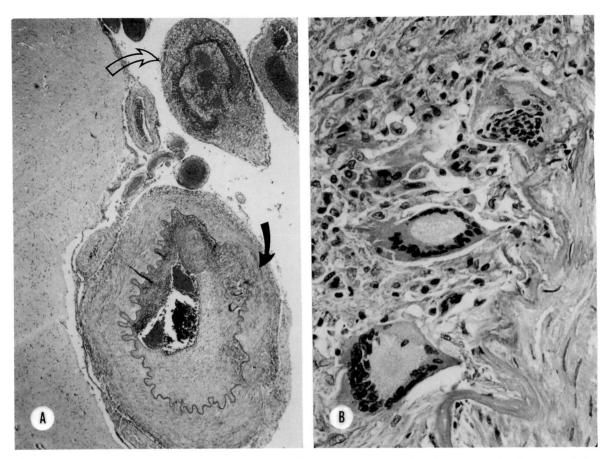

Figure 9.33. A. Coexisting granulomatous (*solid arrow*) and necrotizing (*open arrow*) primary angiitis of the CNS. **B.** Close-up view of the area in **A,** indicated by the solid arrow, to show Langhans and foreign-body type giant cells.

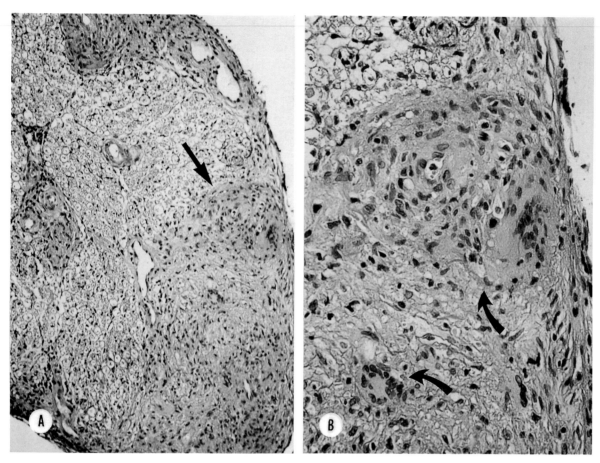

Figure 9.34. A. Granulomatous primary angiitis (*arrow*) in spinal cord biopsy. **B.** Close-up view of giant cell (*arrows*) in the granulomatous angiitis.

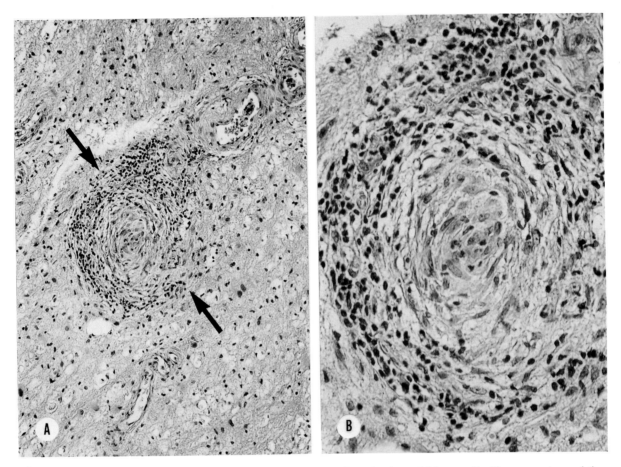

Figure 9.35. A. Lymphocytic primary angiitis (*arrows*) in spinal cord biopsy. **B.** Close-up view of the lymphocytic angiitis without giant cells.

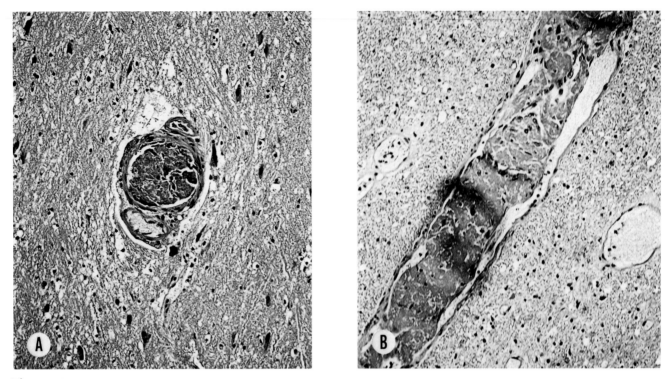

Figure 9.36. Microvascular thromboses in positive brain **(A)** and spinal cord **(B)** biopsies for primary angiitis of the CNS.

Section 3 MISCELLANEOUS RELATED DISORDERS

10. Amyloidosis

Amyloidosis is a clinical disorder characterized by systemic or isolated extracellular deposition of insoluble fibrillar proteins. Amyloidosis is not a single entity but, rather, a diverse family of diseases, of which each member may be identified immunochemically by its unique variety of amyloid protein fibrils and clinically by a distinct syndrome. Amyloid protein can be identified by its nonbranching fibrillar ultrastructure with electron microscopy; by a crossed β pattern on x-ray diffraction; and by an apple-green birefringence on polarized microscopy after Congo red staining of the affected tissue. The amyloid fibril is formed from several and often unrelated proteins or protein fragments with the common ability of assuming the β-pleated sheet structure under appropriate conditions. At present, 17 such amyloidogenic proteins or protein fragments have been characterized by amino acid sequence and, in many cases, complementary DNA also has been established.

CLASSIFICATIONS OF AMYLOIDOSIS

Traditionally, different clinical syndromes of amyloidosis were classified clinically into *primary* (arising de novo) and *secondary* (associated with another clinical disorder); anatomically into *typical* and *atypical* according to organ-tissue involvements; and empirically by its patterns of distribution (Table 10.1). Given the heterogeneity of amyloidosis, variations in and overlapping patterns of the amyloid deposits distribution in different categories were not surprising and the empirical methods of classification became a constant source of confusion.

Within the past two decades, significant developments in immunochemical identification and characterization of different amyloid fibril proteins have made it possible to formulate a rational classification based on the amyloid protein types isolated (Table 10.2). Primary and myeloma-associated types of amyloid are composed of immunoglobulin κ or λ light chains, or fragments thereof, designated as AL amyloid (*A* for amyloid and *L* for light chain). AL amyloid frequently occurs in association with monoclonal gammopathies and, in a significant number of cases, AL amyloid deposition may precede the onset of clinically overt plasma cell dyscrasias.

The amyloid protein associated with a variety of chronic or recurrent inflammatory disorders, such as rheumatoid arthritis and familial Mediterranean fever, and certain malignancies, differs in amino acid se-

quence from immunoglobulins and is named AA amyloid. Its serum precursor, SAA, is a soluble protein and can be isolated with the HDL_3 subclass of lipoproteins. However, there are also reports of AA protein occurring in idiopathic, or, primary amyloidosis.

The amyloid protein of familial amyloidotic polyneuropathy, AF amyloid, has been isolated and identified as consisting of prealbumin; and the isolated cardiac amyloid protein may also be related to this same serum precursor. The amyloid proteins in endocrine tumors are yet again different. To date, at least three distinct types of age-related cardiovascular amyloid proteins have been described: isolated atrial amyloidosis (IAA), senile cardiac amyloidosis (SCA), and senile isolated aortic amyloidosis (SIA).

BIOPSY DIAGNOSIS OF AMYLOIDOSIS

The diagnosis of amyloidosis is made by the demonstration, with an appropriate array of stains, of amyloid deposits in tissue samples obtained by biopsy or needle-aspiration. The reported sensitivity range of these procedures, as reviewed by Hazenberg and van Rijswijk (1994), is as follows: in biopsies, kidney ± 90% (Fig. 10.1), small bowel, duodenum, or stomach ± 90% (Fig.10.2), labial salivary gland ± 85%, and rectum ±80%; all of which exceed the sensitivity of subcutaneous fat needle-aspirate of ± 60% (Fig. 10.3), but the latter has the appeal of being the least invasive procedure. Liver biopsy for the diagnosis of amyloidosis should be avoided if at all possible because of the real risk of uncontrollable hemorrhage as a complication.

The biopsy tissue sections should be cut at least at 5 μm thick and stained with at least two different "amyloid" stains, because none of which, including Congo red, is truly specific for amyloid. The popular choices of pairs are Congo red and methyl violet, Congo red and sulfated alcian blue, or Congo red with thioflavin T or thioflavin F; the thioflavin stained sections require light microscopic examination under ultra-violet light. All Congo red stained sections should be examined in polarized light for birefringence. Immunohistochemical staining with specific monoclonal antibodies is employed to differentiate AA from other amyloid proteins.

The heart and lungs may be involved in systemic amyloidosis, and the heart alone in isolated cardiac amyloidosis. Cardiac amyloidosis may be asymptomatic or an important cause of severe and refractory progressive heart failure and arrhythmia. Cardiac amyloidosis

Table 10.1 Empirical Classifications of Amyloidosis

A. Clinicopathological Classification

1. *Primary Amyloidosis.* Amyloidosis not associated with a known underlying disease, and the amyloid deposits are found predominantly in the heart, lungs, liver, gastrointestinal tract, lymphnodes, skeletal muscle, and skin.

2. *Secondary Amyloidosis.* Amyloidosis associated with a known underlying disease other than multiple myeloma, and the amyloid deposits are found predominantly in the liver, spleen, kidneys, and adrenals.

3. *Tumor-Forming Amyloidosis.* Localized or isolated amyloid deposits in the eyes, upper respiratory tract, urinary bladder, bones, and skin.

4. *Amyloidosis of Multiple Myeloma.* Organ distribution of amyloid deposits resembling that of *primary* amyloidosis.

B. Anatomical Classification

1. *Typical Amyloidosis.* Amyloid deposits in the usual sites (liver, spleen, kidneys, etc.)
   a. Associated with an underlying disease, including multiple myeloma.
   b. Not associated with an underlying disease.

2. *Atypical Amyloidosis.* Amyloid deposits in sites other than those found in typical amyloidosis, and the localized or isolated type.
   a. Associated with an underlying disease, including multiple myeloma.
   b. Not associated with an underlying disease.

C. Patterns of Distribution Classification

1. *Pattern I.* Principal involvement of the tongue, gastrointestinal tract, heart, skeletal and smooth muscles, carpal ligaments, nerves and skin (i.e., resembling the *primary* or *typical* amyloidosis).

2. *Pattern II.* Principal involvement of the liver, spleen, kidneys, and adrenals (i.e., resembling the *secondary* or *atypical* amyloidosis).

3. *Mixed Patterns I and II.*

4. *Localized Pattern.* Amyloid deposits exclusively in a single organ or tissue.

can be reliably diagnosed by endomyocardial biopsies with adequate tissue samples (a minimum of 5 fragments). The pattern of amyloid deposits in the heart may be perifiber (Fig. 10.4), nodular interstitial, vascular (Fig. 10.5), or mixed, and they can be graded semiquantitatively. Cardiac involvement in primary amyloidosis tends to be higher grade and frequently (± 90%) vascular in distribution. The heart with senile cardiac amyloidosis, tends to be lower grade with a predominantly

(± 90%) nodular interstitial pattern of deposits, and rarely (< 5%) vascular in distribution. Lung involvement in amyloidosis may be vascular (Fig. 10.6) or nodular ("amyloidoma"); the former may be a cause of pulmonary hypertension and the latter may mimic neoplastic disease.

Amyloid deposition is ubiquitous and one should expect the unexpected. Involvement of the temporal artery may cause jaw claudication and clinically mimic giant cell (temporal) arteritis.

BIBLIOGRAPHY

Cohen AS: Amyloidosis. *N Engl J Med* 277:522–530; 574–583; 628–638, 1967.

Cooper JH: Selective amyloid staining as a function of amyloid structure: Histochemical analysis of the alkaline Congo red, standardized toluidine blue, and iodine methods. *Lab Invest* 31:232–238, 1974.

Duston MA, Skinner M, Meenan RF, Cohen AS: Sensitivity, specificity, and predictive value of abdominal fat aspiration for the diagnosis of amyloidosis. *Arthritis Rheum* 32:82–85, 1989.

Glenner GG: Amyloid deposits and amyloidosis: The β-fibrilloses. *N Engl J Med* 302:1283–1292; 1333–1343, 1980.

Hachulla E, Janin A, Flipo RM, et al: Labial salivary gland biopsy is a reliable test for the diagnosis of primary and secondary amyloidosis. *Arthritis Rheum* 36:691–697, 1993.

Hawkins PN: Diagnosis and monitoring of amyloidosis. *Bailliére's Clin Rheumatol* 8:635–639, 1994.

Hazenberg BPC, van Rijswijk MH: Clinical and therapeutic aspects of AA amyloidosis. *Bailliére's Clin Rheumatol* 8:661–690, 1994.

Husby G: Classification of amyloidosis. *Bailliére's Clin Rheumatol* 8:503–511, 1994.

Husby G, Araki S, Benditt EP, et al: Nomenclature of amyloid and amyloidosis. *Bull World Health Organ* 71:105–108, 1993.

Isobe T, Osserman EF: Patterns of amyloidosis and their association with plasma cell dyscrasia, monoclonal immunoglobulins and Bence-Jones proteins. *N Engl J Med* 290:473–477, 1974.

Johnson WJ, Lie JT: Pulmonary hypertension and familial Mediterranean fever: A previously unrecognized association. *Mayo Clin Proc* 66:919–925, 1991.

Table 10.2 Immunochemical Classification of Amyloidosis

Clinical Entity	Amyloid Protein	Presumed Precursors
Primary (Idiopathic) Amyloidosis	AL (Aκ and Aλ)	Immunoglobulin light chains or fragments
■ Plasma cell dyscrasias		
■ Macroglobulinemia		
■ Agammaglobulinemia		
■ Lymphoid tumors		
■ Organ-limited (diffuse or focal)		
Secondary (Reactive) Amyloidosis	AA	Serum AA protein
■ Chronic suppurative inflammation		
■ Recurrent inflammation		
■ Hodgkin's disease		
■ Nonlymphoid solid tumors		
■ Familial Mediterranean fever (FMF)		
Heredofamilial Amyloidosis (Excluding FMF)	AF	Prealbumin
■ Familial amyloidotic polyneuropathy		
Endocrinopathic Amyloidosis		
■ Medullary carcinoma of thyroid	AEt	Procalcitonin
■ Islet-cell amyloidosis in type 2 diabetes	AEi	Insulin
Senile Amyloidosis		
■ Cardiac	ASc	Prealbumin
■ Brain ("Congophilic Angiopathy")	ASb	Prealbumin

King LS: Atypical amyloid disease, with observations on a new silver stain for amyloid. *Am J Pathol* 24:1095–1115, 1948.

Kisilevky R, Young ID: Pathogenesis of amyloidosis. *Bailliére's Clin Rheumatol* 8:613–626, 1994.

Kyle RA: Amyloidosis. *Clin Hematol* 11:151–180, 1982.

Kyle RA, Gertz MA: Primary amyloidosis: Clinical and laboratory features in 474 cases. *Semin Hematol* 32:45–59, 1995.

Lie JT: Amyloidosis and amyloid heart disease. *Prim Cardiol* 8(7): 75–92, 1982.

Lie JT: Pathology of amyloidosis and amyloid heart disease. *Applied Pathol* 2:341–356, 1984.

Marenco JL, Sanchez-Burson J, Ruiz-Campos J, et al: Pulmonary amyloidosis and unusual lung involvement in SLE. *Clin Rheumatol* 13:525–527, 1994.

Marhaug G, Dowton SB: Serum amyloid A: An acute phase apolipoprotein and precursor of AA amyloid. *Bailliére's Clin Rheumatol* 8:553–573, 1994.

Maury CPJ: Molecular pathogenesis of β-amyloidosis in Alzheimer's disease and other cerebral amyloidosis. *Lab Invest* 72:4–16, 1995.

Okuda Y, Takasugi K, Oyama T, et al: Amyloidosis in rheumatoid arthritis: Clinical study of 124 histologically proven cases. *Ryumachi* 34:939–946, 1994.

Salvarani C, Gabriel SE, Gertz MA, et al: Primary systemic amyloidosis presenting as giant cell arteritis and polymyalgia rheumatica. *Arthritis Rheum* 37:1621–1626, 1994.

Smith TJ, Kyle RA, Lie JT: Clinical significance of histopathologic patterns of cardiac amyloidosis. *Mayo Clin Proc* 59:547–555, 1984.

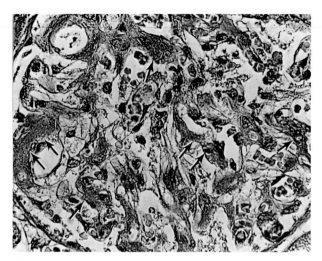

Figure 10.1. Close-up view of glomerular tuft amyloid deposits (*arrows*) in a renal biopsy.

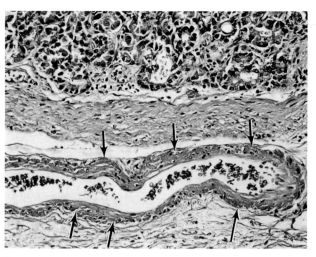

Figure 10.2. Submucosal vascular amyloid deposits (*arrows*) in a gastric mucosal biopsy.

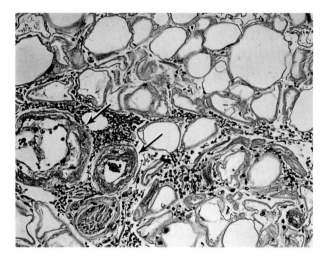

Figure 10.3. Vascular (*arrows*) and periadipocyte amyloid deposits in an abdominal subcutaneous fat needle-aspirate.

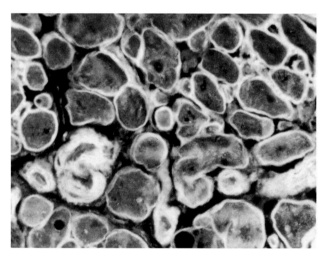

Figure 10.4. Bright rings of perifiber cardiac amyloidosis seen in an endomyocardial biopsy stained with thioflavin-T and examined under ultra-violet light microscopy.

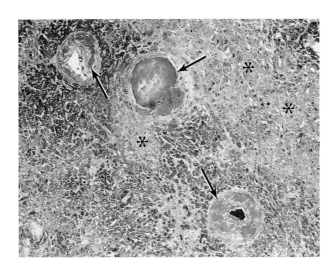

Figure 10.5. Nodular interstitial (*asterisks*) and vascular (*arrows*) cardiac amyloidosis of plasma cell dyscrasia seen in an endomyocardial biopsy.

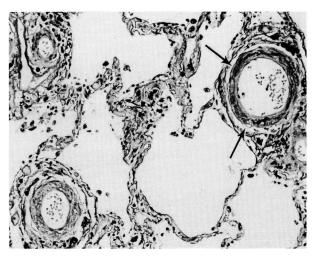

Figure 10.6. Pulmonary hypertension with vascular amyloid deposits (*arrows*) seen in an open lung biopsy of a patient with familial Mediterranean fever.

11. Antiphospholipid Syndromes

PRIMARY, SECONDARY, AND CATASTROPHIC ANTIPHOSPHOLIPID SYNDROMES

Antiphospholipid antibodies (aPL) are a group of closely related immunoglobulin autoantibodies that interact with one or more negatively charged phospholipids measurable by several different laboratory assay systems. The three key members of aPL are reagin, lupus anticoagulant (LA), and anticardiolipin antibodies (aCL).

The aPL may be detectable in a variety of clinical settings; the transient appearance of aPL is almost an universal response to cell injury, infections, malignancies and nonmalignant systemic disease, and as the side effect of certain therapeutic agents. In addition, aPL may be detected in up to 10% of normal populations, and the frequency of detection increases with aging. It is the persistence and elevated levels of circulating aPL that appear to be associated with a variety of clinical disorders that are known collectively as the *antiphospholipid syndrome* (APS).

The first clinical description of APS, though not so named, was probably a case report by Johansson et al. in 1977, with the long title "A peripheral vascular syndrome overlapping with systemic lupus erythematosus: Recurrent venous thrombosis and hemorrhagic capillary proliferation with circulating anticoagulants and false-positive seroreactions for syphilis." In mid-1980s, the clinical syndrome of recurrent venous and/or arterial thrombosis, with or without recurrent fetal loss, thrombocytopenia and/or hemolytic anemia, in patients tested positively for circulating LA, aCL, or both, was initially dubbed "the anticardiolipin syndrome" by Hughes et al., or "the antiphospholipid antibody syndrome" by Harris et al., in 1985. It was later re-named "the antiphospholipid syndrome" by Harris et al. in 1987, with a proposed set of tentative clinical diagnostic criteria (Table 11.1).

The APS comes of age in just one decade. With the probable sole exception of the acquired immunodeficiency syndrome (AIDS), no other clinical entities have attracted greater attention in the biomedical community or figured more prominently in the scientific journals worldwide than APS in the 1980s and 1990s. Although APS was initially encountered in patients with systemic lupus erythematosus (SLE), or a lupus-like disease, it soon became apparent that a considerable number of patients with the syndrome do not have SLE or a lupus-like disease, but may have a wide variety of conditions that include other connective tissue disorders, malig-nancies, infections (including AIDS), or having had prolonged treatment with some drugs known as lupus inducers; these patients have the *secondary* APS. But APS also has been recognized with increasing frequency in the absence of any of the above conditions; the concept of a *primary* APS was introduced by Asherson in 1988, and an exclusion clinical criteria for primary APS also have been formulated (Table 11.2). A subset of primary or secondary APS patients with serious or life-threatening multisystem complications are designated as having the *catastrophic* APS.

CLINICAL MANIFESTATIONS OF ANTIPHOSPHOLIPID SYNDROMES

The clinical distinction between primary and secondary APS is not absolute; there are patients with primary APS who, in time (after as long as 10 years or longer), may develop features of SLE or a lupus-like disease. To date, there is no conclusive evidence that the primary APS differs in any way from secondary APS with regard to the nature of aPL, nor the types, frequency, and outcome of all known complications of the syndrome. The possible exceptions are that valvular heart disease, autoimmune hemolytic anemia, low C4 levels, and neutropenia appear to be somewhat more common in SLE patients with secondary APS than in patients with primary APS. The clinical manifestations of primary and secondary APS are varied and diverse, involving virtually every organ-system in the body, with recurrent arterial and/or venous thrombotic vaso-occlusive disease (VOD) as the common pathogenetic mechanism (Table 11.3). However, the results of antithrombotic therapy in APS patients with VOD is highly variable; some patients respond satisfactorily to oral low-dose aspirin while others require treatment with parenteral fibrinolytic agents, including tissue plasminogen activator. For the majority of both the primary and secondary APS patients, despite adequate anticoagulant therapy, they remain at high risk (compared with controls) of developing further thromboembolic complications.

VASCULITIS IN ANTIPHOSPHOLIPID SYNDROMES, CULPRIT OR CONSORT?

Shortly after APS became established as a recognized entity, a controversy existed on the true nature of the vasculopathy, thrombosis or vasculitis, that is responsi-

Table 11.1 Candidate for the Antiphospholipid Syndrome*

A young person (< 45 yrs) with any of the following:
- More than one episode of unexplained venous thrombosis
- One or more episodes of cerebral or myocardial ischemia, or other arterial thrombotic events (without known risk factors)
- One or more fetal losses in late second or third trimester
- Combination of any of the above, and

High-level positive IgG anticardiolipin antibody test and/or unequivocal positive circulating lupus anticoagulant test

*Modified from Harris EN. *J Rheumatol* 1990;17:733–735

Table 11.2 Exclusion Clinical Criteria for the Primary Antiphospholipid Syndrome (APS)*

The presence of any of these following criteria excludes the diagnosis of APS
- Malar rash
- Discoid rash
- Oral or pharyngeal ulceration, excluding nasal septal ulceration or perforation
- Frank arthritis
- Pleuritis in the absence of pulmonary embolism or left-heart failure
- Pericarditis in the absence of myocardial infarction or uremia
- Proteinuria (> 0.5 g/day) due to immune complex related glomerulonephritis
- Lymphopenia (< 1,000/μl)
- Antibodies to native DNA by immunoassay of *Crithidia* fluorescence
- Anti-extractable nuclear antigen antibodies
- Antinuclear antibodies positive (> 1:320)
- Treatment with any drugs known to induce antiphospholipid antibodies

A followup longer than 5 years after first clinical manifestation is necessary to rule out the subsequent emergence of SLE

*Modified from Piette et al.: *J Rheumatol* 1993;20:1802–1804

ble for the various clinical manifestations of the syndrome. The controversy lingers largely for the following reasons: imprecise usage of terminology; confusion between reactive inflammatory cell infiltrate and a true vasculitis (Fig. 11.1); erroneous acceptance of immune complex deposition in the blood vessel walls as evidence of vasculitis; and, frequently and most importantly, the failure to distinguish between a vasculitis coincidental with and one that is causally related to the APS.

One should be reminded that "vasculopathy" simply means a disorder of the blood vessel from any cause without inference to either the etiology or its morphologic expression, but the term has been loosely and incorrectly used as interchangeable with "vasculitis." Vasculitis is defined as a true inflammatory disease of the blood vessel, artery or vein, with demonstrable structural injury to the vessel wall; the cause of vasculitis may be unknown (*primary* vasculitis) or the vasculitis is a manifestation of one of a diverse variety of existing underlying diseases (*secondary vasculitis*). Likewise, an organized thrombus with neoangiogenesis may also have some reactive cellular infiltrate and has been misinterpreted as a healing or healed vasculitis.

Can vasculitis occur in patients with APS? The answer is an emphatic yes, but the vasculitis is present as a consort. Has the APS been unequivocally shown to be the cause of vasculitis? The answer is an equally emphatic no, and thrombosis is still the culprit of VOD in APS.

A vasculitis may occur in APS patients in two different situations. First, the vasculitis is associated with a known independent underlying disease, such as SLE, coincidental with APS in the same patient. Second, and more rarely, microvascular injury manifesting as capillaritis may coexist with APS in a patient. Capillaritis is more a quasivasculitis than true vasculitis. Capillary is a single-cell layer vascular loop lined by the endothelium, perhaps with a pericyte but without vascular smooth muscle cells externally. Unlike arteries and veins, or arterioles and venules, inflammatory injury to a capillary (capillaritis) cannot be identified histologically in the usual manner by the cellular infiltrate in and the structural injury to the blood vessel wall. The diagnosis of a capillaritis is inferred by the "spilling" of inflammatory cell infiltrate, with granulocyte karyorrhexis and erythrocyte extravasation over the injured capillary network; the affected capillary loops may be damaged beyond recognition. In the kidney, capillaritis appears as necrotizing glomerulonephritis and, in the lung, as pulmonary capillaritis associated with diffuse alveolar hemorrhage (Fig. 11.2).

BIOPSY DIAGNOSIS IN THE ANTIPHOSPHOLIPID SYNDROMES

The biopsy diagnosis in the APS patients has a two-fold objective; the first is to determine if the APS is primary or secondary, and the second is to confirm thromboem-

Table 11.3 Sequelae of Recurrent Arterial and/or Venous Thrombosis in APS

Thromboembolic Disease	Clinical Manifestations
Head and neck, eyes, and central nervous system	Transient ischemic attacks, stroke, Sneddon syndrome, acute ischemic encephalopathy, multiinfarct dementia, retinal artery/arteriolar thrombosis, visual disturbances
Heart, valvular and mural endocardium	Myocardial ischemia/infarction, Libman-Sacks endocarditis mural thrombosis, brady-tachyarrhythmia
Lungs	Pulmonary thromboembolism, pulmonary hypertension, capillaritis and diffuse alveolar hemorrhage
Vena cavae and tributaries	Superior and inferior vena cava syndromes
Aorta and limb branches	Aortic arch syndrome, limb claudication and gangrene
Mesentery	Visceral angina, ischemic bowel disease and infarction
Liver	Hepatic or portal vein thrombosis, portal hypertension, hepatic infarction, Budd-Chiari syndrome, hepatic regenerative nodular hyperplasia
Kidneys	Renal artery and/or vein thrombosis, infarcts, renovascular hypertension, thrombotic glomerular microangiopathy
Adrenals	Central vein thrombosis, hemorrhage, with or without infarcts, Addison's disease, hypoadrenalism
Skin	Rash, palpable purpura, livido reticularis, cutaneous ulcers, digital gangrene
Placenta	Arterial/venous/capillary thrombosis, recurrent fetal deaths

bolism as the basis of VOD in APS, both of which directly affect the decision making process in the choice of therapy.

To determine the frequency and types of VOD in APS, Bacharach and Lie (1992) reviewed the records of 102 consecutive patients, 72 females and 30 males ranging in age from 14 to 79 years (mean, 46), whose sera tested positively for IgG and/or IgM anticardiolipin antibodies. Lupus anticoagulant was detectable in 17 (25%) of 67 patients tested. VOD was identified in 80 (78%) of these 102 patients, of whom, 65 (81%) had primary APS and 15 (19%) had secondary APS. A variety of VODs were found: together, 27 (34%) had cerebrovascular VOD; 17 (21%) each recurrent venous thrombosis or fetal loss; 11 (14%) arterial thrombosis other than that of the coronary artery; 5 (6%) visceral infarction; 3 (4%) coronary artery thrombosis; and none had vasculitis (Table 11.4). Major nonfatal complications of APS-associated VOD (excluding the 17 recurrent fetal loss) occurred in 34 patients: 14 had stroke (Fig. 11.3); 7 pulmonary embolism or thrombosis (Fig. 11.4); 4 below-knee amputation (Fig. 11.5), and 2 cutaneous thrombosis (Fig. 11.6); 3 pulmonary hypertension (Fig. 11.7); 3 myocardial infarction (Figs. 11.8 and 11.9); 2 bowel resection (Fig. 11.10); and 1 nephrectomy for infarction preceded by thrombotic glomerular microangiopathy (Fig. 11.11). Three patients in this series of 80 with VOD subsequently died of catastrophic APS from multi-system recurrent arterial and venous

Table 11.4 Types of Vaso-Occlusive Disease in 80 APS Patients

Clinical Manifestations	Primary APS	Secondary APS
Cerebrovascular disease	22	5
Recurrent fetal losses	14	3
Recurrent venous thrombosis	14	3
Recurrent arterial thrombosis	7	4
Visceral infarction	5	0
Coronary artery thrombosis	3	0
Total	65	15

thrombosis within a 5-year followup period; two had Libman-Sacks endocarditis (Fig. 11.12).

CONCLUSION

Whether the vasculopathy in APS is thrombotic or vasculitic should have biopsy confirmation where possible. The distinction is important not only for unravelling the pathogenesis of VOD in APS but also for selecting the appropriate form of drug treatment. A diagnosis of vasculitis in secondary APS would call for treatment with corticosteroids and cytotoxic agents, which are not without serious side effects to the patients. The same powerful and potentially toxic drugs are clearly quite ineffectual in preventing or treating APS-associated thrombosis which, on the other hand, has been known to respond to the lowly and inexpensive aspirin.

BIBLIOGRAPHY

Alarcón-Segovia D, Cardiel MH, Reyes E: Antiphospholipid arterial vasculopathy. *J Rheumatol* 16:762–767, 1989.

Asherson RA: The catastrophic antiphospholipid syndrome. *J Rheumatol* 19:508–512, 1992.

Asherson RA, Cervera R: The antiphospholipid syndrome: A syndrome in evolution. *Ann Rheum Dis* 51: 147–150, 1992.

Asherson RA, Cervera R: Review: Antiphospholipid antibodies and the lung. *J Rheumatol* 22:62–66, 1995.

Asherson RA, Khamashta MA, Ordi-Ros J, et al: The "primary" antiphospholipid syndrome: Major clinical and serological features. *Medicine* 68:366–374, 1989.

Bacharach JM, Lie JT: The prevalence of vascular occlusive disease associated with the antiphospholipid syndrome. *Int Angiol* 11:51–56, 1992.

Bacharach JM, Lie JT: Lupus anticoagulant, anticardiolipin antibodies, and the antiphospholipid syndrome. In Frolich ED, Cooke JP (eds). *Current Management of Hypertensive and Vascular Diseases.* St. Louis, Mosby-Year Book, 1992:355–360.

Bansal AS, Hogan PG, Gibbs H, Frazer IH: Familial primary antiphospholipid antibody syndrome. *Arthritis Rheum* 39:705–706, 1996.

Bick RL (ed): Antiphospholipid Syndromes. *Semin Thromb Hemost* 20:1–132, 1994.

Castañón C, Amigo M-C, Bañales JL, et al: Ocular vaso-occlusive disease in primary antiphospholipid syndrome. *Ophthalmology* 102:256–262, 1995.

Cervera R, Asherson RA, Lie JT: Clinicopathologic correlations of the antiphospholipid syndrome. *Semin Arthritis Rheum* 24:262–272, 1995.

Cohen MG, Lui SF: Multiple complications of the antiphospholipid syndrome with apparent response to aspirin therapy. *J Rheumatol* 19:803–806, 1992.

Font J, López-Soto A, Cervera R, et al: The "primary antiphospholipid syndrome": Antiphospholipid antibody pattern and clinical features of a series of 23 patients. *Autoimmunity* 9:69–75, 1991.

Ford SE, Ford PM: The cardiovascular pathology of antiphospholipid antibodies: An illustrative case and review of the literature. *Cardiovasc Pathol* 4:111–122, 1995.

Gertner E, Lie JT: Pulmonary capillaritis, alveolar hemorrhage and recurrent microvascular thrombosis in primary antiphospholipid syndrome. *J Rheumatol* 20:1224–1228, 1993.

Goldberger E, Elder RC, Schwartz RA, Phillips PE: Vasculitis in the antiphospholipid syndrome. *Arthritis Rheum* 35:569–572, 1992.

Harris EN: Syndrome of the black swan. *Br J Rheumatol* 26:324–326, 1987.

Harris EN: Antiphospholipid antibodies. *Br J Haematol* 74:1–9, 1990.

Harris EN, Baguley E, Asherson RA, Hughes GRV: Clinical and serological features of the "antiphospholipid syndrome." (*abstract*) *Br J Rheumatol* 26:324–326, 1987.

Harris EN, Gharavi AE, Hughes GRV: Antiphospholipid antibodies. *Clin Rheum Dis* 11:591–609, 1985.

Hughes GRV: The anticardiolipin syndrome. *Clin Exp Rheumatol* 3:285–286, 1985.

Hughes GRV: The antiphospholipid syndrome: Ten years on. *Lancet* 342:341–344, 1993.

Khamashta MA, Hughes GRV: Antiphospholipid antibodies and antiphospholipid syndrome. *Curr Opin Rheumatol* 7:389–394, 1995.

Johansson EA, Niemi KM, Mustakallio KK: A peripheral vascular syndrome overlapping with systemic lupus erythematosus: Recurrent venous thrombosis and hemorrhagic capillary proliferation with circulating anticoagulants and false-positive seroreactions for syphilis. *Dermatologia* 155:257–263, 1977.

Lie JT: Vasculopathy in the antiphospholipid syndrome: Thrombosis or vasculitis, or both? *J Rheumatol* 16: 713–715, 1989.

Lie JT: The distinction between vasculitis coincidental with and one that is causally related to the antiphospholipid syndrome. *Arthritis Rheum* 35:1540, 1992.

Lie JT: Vasculitis in the antiphospholipid syndrome: Culprit or consort? *J Rheumatol* 21:397–399, 1994.

Lie JT: Nomenclature and classification of vasculitis: Plus ça change, plus c'est la même chose. *Arthritis Rheum* 37:181–186, 1994.

Lie JT: Pathology of the antiphospholipid syndrome. In Asherson, RA, Cervera R, Piette J-C, Shoenfeld Y (eds). *The Antiphospholipid Syndrome.* Boca Raton, Florida, CRC Press 1996:89–104.

Lie JT, Kobayashi S, Tokano Y, Hashimoto H: Systemic and cerebral vasculitis coexisting with disseminated coagulopathy in systemic lupus erythematosus associated with antiphospholipid syndrome. *J Rheumatol* 22:2173–2176, 1995.

Mackworth-Young CG: Antiphospholipid antibodies and disease. (The Michael Mason Prize Essay, 1994) *Br J Rheumatol* 34:1009–1030, 1995.

Mackworth-Young CG, Loizou S, Wolport MJ, et al: Primary antiphospholipid syndrome: Features of patients with raised anticardiolipin antibodies and no other disorders. *Ann Rheum Dis* 48:362–367, 1989.

Muir KW: Anticardiolipin antibodies and cardiovascular disease. *J Roy Soc Med* 88:433–436, 1995.

Mujic F, Cuadrado MJ, Lloyd M, et al: Primary antiphospholipid syndrome evolving into systemic lupus erythematosus. *J Rheumatol* 22:1589–1592, 1995.

Out HJ, van Vliet M, de Groot PG, Derksen RHWM: Prospective study of fluctuations of lupus anticoagulant activity and anticardiolipin antibody titre in patients with systemic lupus erythematosus. *Ann Rheum Dis* 51:353–357, 1992.

Pérez RE, McClendon JR, Lie JT: Primary antiphospholipid syndrome with multiorgan arterial and venous thrombosis. *J Rheumatol* 19:1289–1292, 1992.

Piette J-C, Cacoub P, Wechsler B: Renal manifestations of the antiphospholipid syndrome. *Semin Arthritis Rheum* 23:357–366, 1994.

Piette J-C, Wechsler B, Frances C, et al: Systemic lupus erythematosus and the antiphospholipid syndrome. *J Rheumatol* 19:1835–1837, 1992.

Piette J-C, Wechsler B, Frances C, et al: Exclusion criteria for primary antiphospholipid syndrome. *J Rheumatol* 20:1802–1803, 1993.

Rocca PV, Siegel LB, Cupps TR: The concomitant expression of vasculitis and coagulopathy: Synergy for marked tissue ischemia. *J Rheumatol* 21:556–560, 1994.

Sandoval J, Amigo M-C, Barragan R, et al: Primary antiphospholipid syndrome presenting as chronic thromboembolic pulmonary hypertension. *J Rheumatol* 23:772–775, 1996.

Tomer Y, Kessler A, Eyal A, et al: Superior vena cava syndrome in a patient with antiphospholipid antibody syndrome. *J Rheumatol* 18:95–97, 1991.

Yokoi K, Hosoi E, Akaike M, et al: Takayasu's arteritis associated with antiphospholipid antibodies: Report of two cases. *Angiology* 47:315–319, 1996

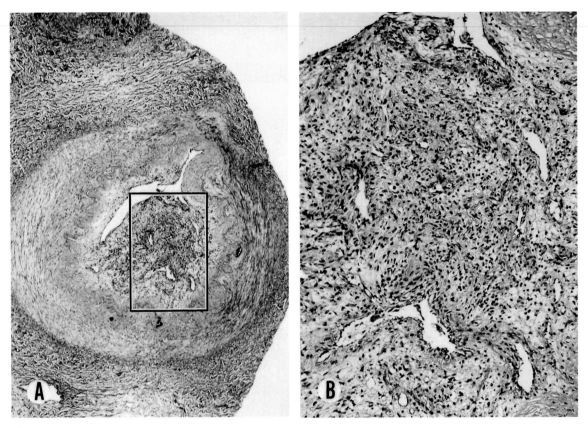

Figure 11.1. Low **(A)** and high **(B)** magnification views of organized thrombus in an artery with neoangiogenesis and residual reactive inflammatory cell infiltrate (*boxed area in A*) that could be and has been misinterpreted as a "healed vasculitis" in APS by some observers.

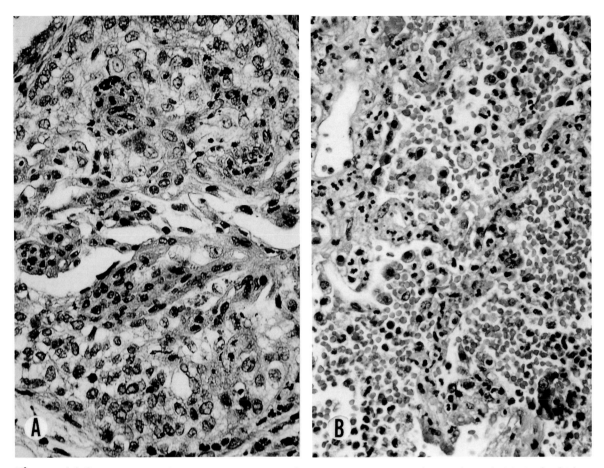

Figure 11.2. Microvascular injury in APS manifesting as necrotizing glomerulonephritis in the kidney **(A)** and as pulmonary capillaritis with diffuse alveolar hemorrhage in the lung **(B)**.

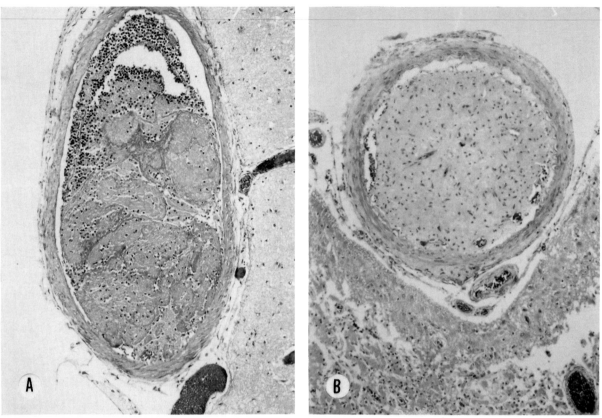

Figure 11.3. APS-associated recurrent vaso-occlusive disease in a patient with stroke, clinically mimicking CNS angiitis. Brain biopsy shows both recent (**A**) and old, organized (**B**) thrombi, and no evidence of vasculitis.

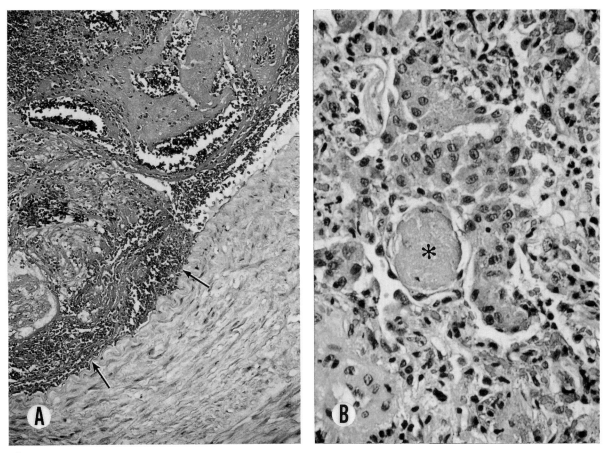

Figure 11.4. Left upper lobectomy specimen in an APS patient with pulmonary infarct shows adherent thrombus (*arrows*) in a primary branch of the left pulmonary artery **(A)** as well as evidence of microvascular thrombosis (*asterisk*) in the left upper lobe lung parenchyma **(B).**

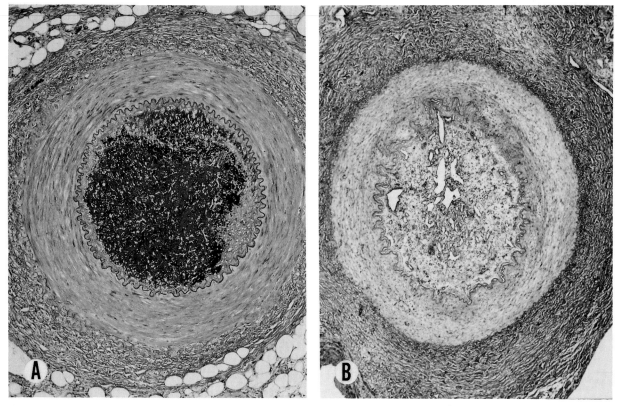

Figure 11.5. Recent (**A**) and old, organized (**B**), recurrent thrombosis in a lower limb artery free of atherosclerosis of a 44-year-old woman with primary APS that resulted in gangrene and a below-knee amputation.

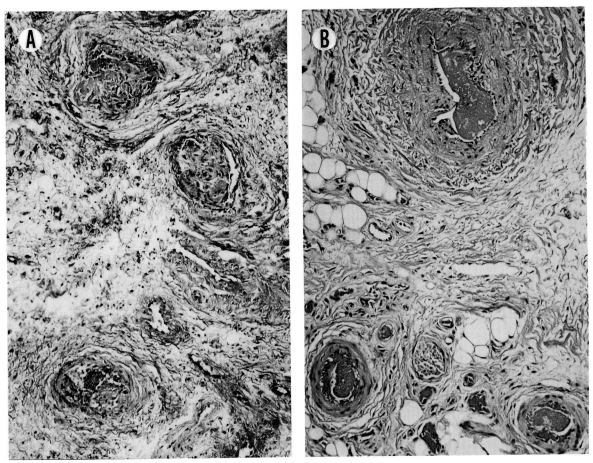

Figure 11.6. Recurrent old **(A)** and recent **(B)** cutaneous small-vessel thrombosis as the cause of livido reticularis and nonhealing skin ulcers.

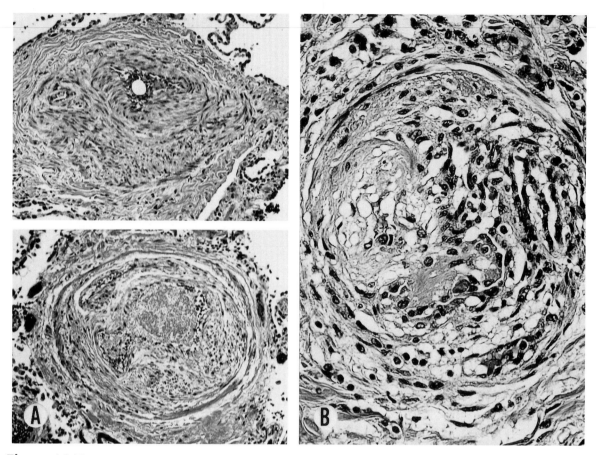

Figure 11.7. Thromboembolic pulmonary hypertension with old, organized (*above*) and recent (*below*) occlusive thrombi (**A**); and Plexogenic pulmonary hypertension (**B**) in APS patients.

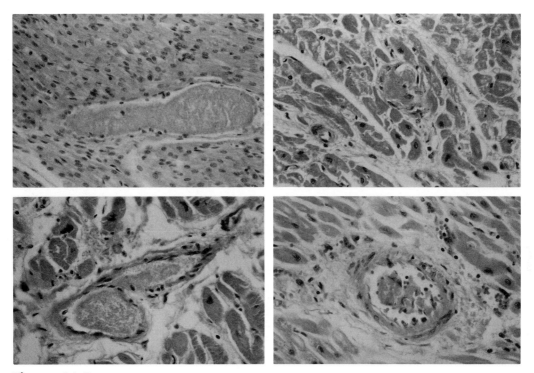

Figure 11.8. A panel of four endomyocardial biopsies with the unexpected findings of microvascular thrombosis in three APS patients presenting with unexplained heart failure.

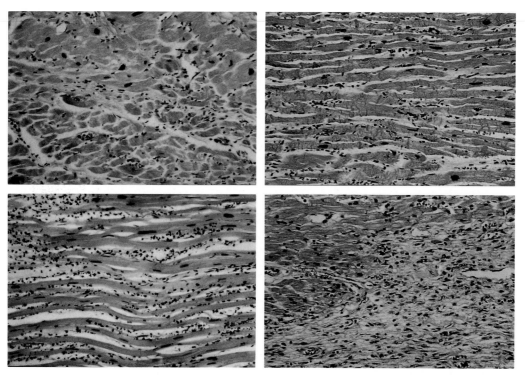

Figure 11.9. A panel of four endomyocardial biopsies showing myocardial infarcts of different histologic ages: hyperacute, within 6 to 9 hours (*upper two*); acute, within 48 hours (*left lower*); and healing, within 3 weeks (*right lower*); in three APS patients with unexplained heart failure.

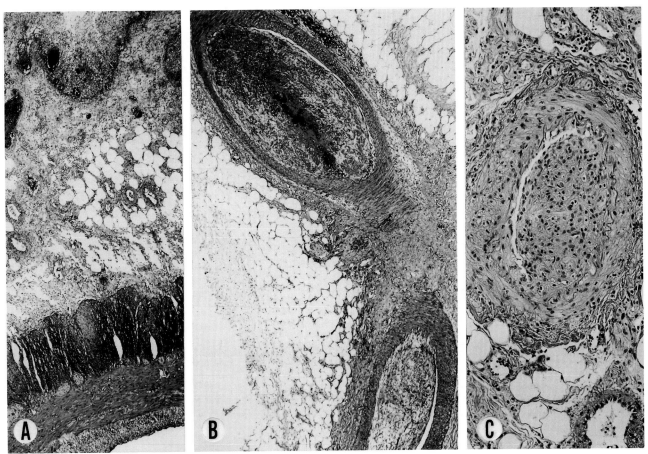

Figure 11.10. Ischemic bowel disease in an APS patient with acute infarction **(A)**, due to recent **(B)** and old **(C)** mesenteric thrombotic vaso-occlusive disease.

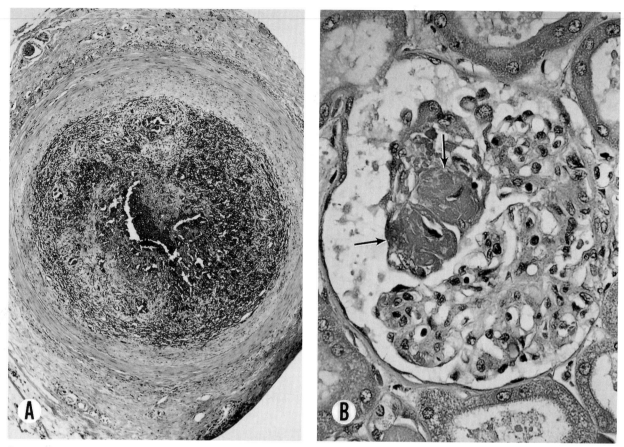

Figure 11.11. Thrombosis in a renal artery free of atherosclerosis **(A)** and thrombotic (*arrows*) glomerular microangiopathy **(B)** in a 33-year-old APS patient who underwent a nephrectomy for infarction one year after progressive renal failure of unknown cause clinically.

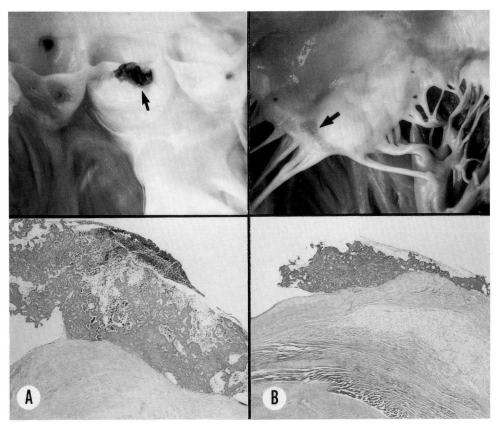

Figure 11.12. One of the three patients, a 48-year-old woman with APS, in whom an earlier endomyocardial biopsy had shown microvascular thrombosis later died of myocardial infarction with aortic **(A)** and mitral **(B)** noninfective thrombotic (Libman-Sacks) endocarditis. Note the grossly normal heart valves (*above*) and the bland fibrin-platelets thrombotic vegetations on the heart valves (*below*).

12. Behçet's Disease

ALL ABOUT BEHÇET'S DISEASE

Behçet syndrome, or Behçet's disease (BD), is one of the oldest maladies known to mankind. According to Aryeh Feigenbaum (1956), a description of the clinical triad of relapsing uveitis with recurrent oral and genital ulceration can be found in the Hippocratic third book of endemic disease. The clinical syndrome, however, was first described in the modern era by Hulûsi Behçet (1889–1948), a Turkish professor of dermatology, who published his observations on two patients in a German-language journal, in 1937. The etiology of BD remains elusive today, and we still rely on the disease pattern recognition for the diagnosis of BD, based on the array of clinical features that Hippocrates found: "Many had their mouth affected with aphthous ulcerations. There were also many defluxations about the genital parts and ulcerations, boils (phymata), externally and internally about the groins."

BD is probably an autoimmune rheumatic disease-related disorder, the likely pathogenetic mechanisms include possibly B-cell mediated autoantibodies with depression of T-cells or an Arthus-type phenomenon involving immune complexes. Because of its remarkable diversity in clinical manifestations, BD is of interest to not only dermatologists and ophthalmologists but also to physicians of virtually every other known subspecialty, as a systemic disease that spares no organ in the body human (Table 12.1). There has been a steadily growing clinical interest in BD over the past four decades; for example, there were only 5 BD citations in the 1955 *Index Medicus,* but the number has risen to 18 in 1965, 48 in 1975, 141 in 1985, and to an estimated more than 500 in 1995. The First International Symposium (or Conference) on Behçet's disease was held in Rome in 1966, and the Seventh is being held in Tunis, Tunisia, in October of 1996.

BD occurs worldwide with a reported patient age distribution that ranges from 6 to 72 years (mean, 24), and the male:female gender ratio from 0.49:1 to 4.9:1, in several major population studies. Moreover, occasional fetal and neonatal cases born to mothers known to have BD also have been described. A number of factors account for the difficulty of estimating the worldwide prevalence of BD, but principally because of the lack of uniform diagnostic criteria adopted by the divergent geographic patient population studies. Reported data on prevalence vary greatly. In most areas of Japan, the esti-mated prevalence of BD per 100,000 is 10, but in the northern island Hokkaido district it is 13.3. The prevalence of BD in most of the Middle-East and the Mediterranean littoral countries equals at least to that in Japan. One suggestion was that the disorder occurs along the length of the old silk routes, but how might the disease have spread from mainland Asia to Japan remains unclear. The prevalence of BD in the United States has been estimated to be 4 to 6 per 100,000, and it is only 0.64 per 100,000 in northern England.

DIAGNOSTIC CRITERIA FOR BEHÇET'S DISEASE

Almost any tissue and organs may be affected by BD, though with vastly different frequencies (Table 12.2); generally, oral ulcers are the most common and appear first, next the cutaneous lesions, followed by ocular, genital, and musculoskeletal involvements. Neurologic and vascular lesions usually evolve later but they may occasionally be the first manifestation of BD, or, indeed, become the major cause of morbidity and mortality of the disease. Association of BD with the B5 and B51 histocompatibility antigen is well known; this association becomes more tenuous further north in Europe and in North America. Retinal complications are more common in the first two years of the disease in B5-positive males and may rapidly become bilateral.

A number of clinical diagnostic criteria for BD have been proposed over the past several decades. The criteria proposed at the 1977 International Symposium on Behçet's Disease held in Istanbul (O'Duffy, 1978) were simple and practical (Table 12.3). The presence of three or more of the seven Istanbul criteria, provided one of these is recurrent oral ulcers, is sufficient for a definite clinical diagnosis of BD; otherwise, the diagnosis of BD is only tentative. However, the self-limiting and common aphthous stomatitis and vulvitis in adolescent females should not be labeled BD. Other clinical entities to be considered in the differential diagnoses include Crohn's disease, herpes simplex infections, and various causes of aseptic meningitis. But after 1990, all previously proposed diagnostic criteria are supplanted by The International Group (ISG) for Behçet's Disease Criteria (Table 12.4). There were two recent independent studies designed to validate the ISG criteria for Behçet's disease, one found a sensitivity of 0.90 and

133

Table 12.1 Clinical Presentations of Behçet's Disease Pertaining to Different Disciplines*

Dermatologist	*Ophthalmologist*	*Neurologist*
Erythema nodosum	Iritis	Strokes, TIA
Oro-genital ulcers	Hypopyon	Meningoencephalitis
Papules/pustules	Retinal vasculitis	Cerebral thrombophlebitis
Blisters	Optic disk edema	Cranial nerve palsy
Purpura	Panophthalmitis	Brain stem ataxia
Dermatographia	Optic neuropathy	Transverse myelitis
Phlebitis	Retinal vein thrombosis	Confusion, dementia
Gastroenterologist	*Rheumatologist*	*Gynecologist/Venereologist*
Oral/bowel/anal ulcers	Synovitis	Genital ulcers
Ischemic bowel disease	Seronegative arthritis	
Colitis, proctitis	Vasculitis	
Regional enteritis		
Splenomegaly		
Chest Physician	*Hematologist/Immunologist*	*Cardiologist/Vascular Physician*
Superior vena cava syndrome	Needle stick hyperreactivity	Thrombophlebitis
Pleuritis/pleural effusion	HLA B5, B12, B27, B51	Arterial/venous thrombosis
Pulmonary aneurysm/vasculitis	↑ Globulins & complements	Myocarditis/endocarditis
Pulmonary capillaritis	↑ C-reactive protein	Pericarditis/effusion
Pulmonary infarction	↑ ESR	Arterial aneurysms
Diffuse alveolar hemorrhage	Immune complex deposition	Peripheral vascular disease
Hemoptysis	Cryoglobulinemia	Vasculitis

*Modified from James DG, Spiteri MA. Behçet's disease. *Ophthalmology* 1982;89:1279–1284.

specificity of 0.95 (O'Neil et al. 1994), and the other (Ferraz et al. 1995), 0.95 and 1.00, respectively.

BIOPSY DIAGNOSIS OF BEHÇET'S DISEASE

While the majority of patients with BD, when suspected clinically, are diagnosed with the ISG criteria, biopsies are helpful when the disease is unsuspected or presents with unusual features. Thrombosis, vascular inflammatory processes including large- and small-vessel vasculitis, and recurrent or multiple arterial aneurysmal disease form the pathologic basis of the clinical manifestations in the vast majority of BD patients. Biopsy diagnosis of BD in accessible tissue samples from the symptomatic sites does not rely on the pathognomonic features, of which there are none, but on changes compatible with or are known to occur in BD.

Mucocutaneous and Small-Vessel Vasculitic Lesions

Recurrent aphthous stomatitis, *sine qua non* of BD, commonly occurs on the lips, gingiva, buccal mucosa,

tongue and, less often, the palate, tonsils and pharynx, may be a single lesion or in clusters, individually 2 to 10 mm in diameter, with a central grayish yellow base surrounded by a discrete erythematous halo. Microscopically, the lesion shows eroded epidermis and a fibrin-covered ulcer floor with an intense mixed-cell infiltrate (Fig.12.1). Cutaneous leukocytoclastic vasculitis or lymphocytic vasculitis occurs in 20 to 40% of BD patients but, of course, neither is etiologically specific for BD (Fig. 12.2); nor is the erythema nodosum-like subcutaneous lesions associated with the delayed-type hypersensitivity reaction. Similarly, a systemic polyarteritis-type necrotizing vasculitis may be seen in a muscle biopsy of BD patients suspected to have inflammatory myopathy (Fig. 12.3). The vasculitis may be so severe as to require plasma exchange treatment.

Gastrointestinal Lesions

Any part of the gastrointestinal tract may be affected in BD, with mucosal ulceration as the predominant lesions. Ischemic bowel diseases, with or without frank infarction, and aseptic pancreatitis, have been attributed to gastrointestinal vasculitis (Fig. 12.4) or vascular amy-

Table 12.2. Behçet's Disease: Major and Minor Clinical Features and Frequency*

Clinical Features	Frequency (%)
MAJOR	
Oral ulcers	99
Eye lesions: anterior uveitis (hypopyon-iritis), posterior uveitis, chorioretinitis, optic nerve atrophy	90
Skin lesions: erythema nodosum, thrombophlebitis, acneiform eruptions, hyperreactivity (needle-stick pathergy test)	85
Genital ulcerations: primarily scrotum and vulva; also penis, perineum, perianal and vaginal mucosa	67
MINOR	
Articular manifestations: arthralgia, arthritis (large joints), myalgia, fibrositis	50
Gastrointestinal manifestations: abdominal pain, melena, inflammatory and ischemic bowel disease	50
Vascular manifestations: arterial and/or venous thrombosis, systemic or pulmonary arterial aneurysms, large- and small-vessel vasculitis with or without thrombosis	28†
Central nervous system manifestations: meningoencephalitis, sensory and motor neuropathy, psychologic changes	15
Epididymitis (in male patients)	10

*Modified from Shimizu et al. *Semin Arthritis Rheum* 1979; 8:223–260.
†Turkish patients, from Koç et al. *J Rheumatol* 1992;19:402–410.

loidosis (Fig. 12.5). Of interest are the different frequencies of these lesions in geographically different patient populations. Gastrointestinal manifestations are uncommon in Turkish BD patients compared with their Japanese and Anglo-Saxon counterparts, but the reverse is true for amyloidosis in BD.

Renal Manifestations

In contrast to genitourinary involvement, renal manifestations of BD are relatively uncommon. Mild abnormal urinalysis, such as proteinuria and/or microhematuria, have been reported to occur in 20% of BD patients in an Israeli series. In renal biopsies of BD patients with renal function impairment, both the diffuse proliferative and

Table 12.3 Behçet's Disease: The Istanbul Diagnostic Criteria*

1. Recurrent aphthous ulcers
2. Recurrent genital ulcers
3. Uveitis (anterior or posterior)
4. Vasculitis (large and small vessels)
5. Synovitis, arthritis (usually large-joint and seronegative)
6. Meningoencephalitis
7. Cutaneous hyperreactivity (positive pathergy test)

*The first criterion plus two others are required for a definite clinical diagnosis of Behçet's disease.

focal necrotizing-type glomerulonephritis (Fig. 12.6) have been observed. Circulating immune complex deposits, when sought, were present in the majority of these renal biopsies.

Cardiovascular Manifestations

Cardiac lesions are also relatively uncommon in BD. Pericardial disease is usually seen during the acute exacerbations of the disease, but has little clinical

Table 12.4 International Study Group Diagnostic Criteria for Behçet's Disease*

Recurrent Oral Ulceration
   Minor aphthous, major aphthous, or herpetiform ulceration observed by a physician or reliably reported by patient, which recurred at least three times in one 12-month period

Plus two of the following
Recurrent Genital Ulceration
   Genital ulceration or scarring, especially males, observed by a physician or reliably reported by patient
Eye Lesions
   Anterior uveitis, posterior uveitis, or cells in vitreous on slit lamp examination; or retinal vasculitis observed by ophthalmologist
Skin Lesions
   Erythema nodosum-like lesions observed by a physician or reliably reported by patient; pseudofolliculitis; papulopustular lesions; or acneiform nodules in post-adolescent patients not on corticosteroid treatment
Positive Pathergy Test
   Test performed with oblique insertion of a 20-gauge or smaller-caliber needle under sterile conditions; reaction to be read by a physician at 24–48 hrs

*Modified from International Study Group for Behçet's Disease. *Lancet* 1990;335:1078–1080.

consequences. Myocarditis and aortic or mitral valve endocarditis have greater clinical significance, but are seldom diagnosed except in an endomyocardial biopsy for heart failure of unexplained origin (Fig. 12.7), and in tissue obtained at surgery for valvular insufficiency or, more rarely, stenosis (Fig. 12.8). Myocarditis and endocarditis in BD may be suspected clinically by the presence of a cardiac murmur, gallop rhythm, ventricular dysfunction, or electrocardiographic changes. A rare aneurysm of the sinus of Valsalva associated with severe aortic regurgitation in BD also has been described.

Although vascular lesions are not included in the ISG Criteria for the diagnosis of BD, up to 25–35% of patients develop arterial and/or venous large-vessel complications; in the former, it is the aneurysmal disease and, in the latter, the thrombosis that predominates. Koç et al. (1992) have reviewed the world literature between 1967 and 1990, and they identified 728 reported cases of large-vessel lesions in BD: 49 were arterial, 181 were venous, and 498 were combined arterial and venous involvement. Antiphospholipid antibodies are detectable in 20 to 30% of patients with BD, and their presence is a predictor of the propensity for recurrent arterial and/or venous thrombosis. As has been noted above, small-vessel vasculitis is common and, to which, many systemic manifestations of BD may be attributed (Figs. 12.1 to 12.4).

Pulmonary Manifestations

Various nonspecific pulmonary lesions occur in BD, some are attributable to complications of terminal events. Autopsy studies have described fibrotic stenosis of the small bronchi and bronchioles with localized emphysematous changes. However, BD may be the only known acquired disorder uniquely associated with multiple pulmonary aneurysms, usually preceded by thromboangiitis of the large and small pulmonary arteries, which is a form of pulmonary vasculitis, and the open lung biopsy findings suggest that the thrombosis is recurrent and episodic (Figs. 12.9 and 12.10). The patients often have coexisting peripheral thrombophlebitis, and this combination is clinically and pathologically indistinguishable from the Hughes-Stovin syndrome (segmental pulmonary artery aneurysms with peripheral venous thrombosis). Rupture of pulmonary artery aneurysms with massive hemoptysis, although uncommon, is a leading cause of sudden unexpected death in BD patients; and the hemoptysis may be the first and unsuspected manifestation of BD.

Synovial and Articular Manifestations

A widely divergent incidence of joint disease in BD has been reported, ranging from 5 to 75% depending on the diagnostic criteria. Synovitis may affect up to 50% of BD patients at some time during the course of their disease. The synovitis may be asymmetric, and the arthritis is usually of the oligo- or monoarticular nondeforming type most commonly affecting the knee joints. A synovial biopsy is seldom indicated in BD, but if carried out, it shows a nongranulomatous acute synovitis with neoangiogenesis, fibrin deposits, and a mixed-cell but predominantly lymphoplasmacytic inflammatory infiltrate (Fig. 12.11). In a comparative study by light and electron microscopic examinations of the synovitis in BD and rheumatoid arthritis patients, Gibson et al. (1981) failed to demonstrate any clearly distinguishing morphologic features, but immunofluorescence microscopy indicated that the consistent IgG deposition in the synovium may be characteristic of BD.

Neurological Manifestations

Neurological manifestations of BD occur in 10 to 30% of the patients and they include an organic confusional state, a meningomyelitic illness, and brain stem syndrome. In autopsy studies, intracranial venous thromboses of the sigmoid, dural, superior sagittal and transverse sinuses are the most common pathologic finding. A brain biopsy in BD patients with neurologic symptoms is performed occasionally to exclude other disorders, such as primary angiitis or intravascular lymphomatosis of the CNS. The biopsy may show nonspecific interstitial and perivascular lymphocytic infiltrate with microvascular fibrin thrombi and, rarely, a small-vessel vasculitis (Fig. 12.12); such findings cannot be differentiated from those seen in patients with CNS lupus or CNS Wegener's granulomatosis without careful clinical correlation.

BIBLIOGRAPHY

Al-Dalaan A, Al-Balaa S, Ali AM, et al: Budd-Chiari syndrome in association with Behçet's disease. *J Rheumatol* 18:622–626, 1991.

Bang D, Honma T, Saito T, et al: The pathogenesis of vascular changes in erythema nodosum-like lesions of Behçet's syndrome: An electron microscopic study. *Hum Pathol* 18:1172–1179, 1987.

Barbas CV, de Carvalho CRR, Delmonte VC, et al: Behçet's disease: A rare case of simultaneous pulmonary and cerebral involvement. *Am J Med* 85: 576–578, 1988.

Bartlett ST, McCarthy WJ III, Palmer AS, et al: Multiple aneurysms in Behçet's disease. *Arch Surg* 123:1004–1008, 1988.

Behçet H: Über rezidivierende aphthöse, durch ein Virus verursachte Geschwüre am Mund, am Auge und an den Genitalien. *Dermatol Wochenschr* 105: 1152–1157, 1937.

Chajek T, Fainaru M: Behçet's disease: Report of 41 cases and a review of the literature. *Medicine* 54: 179–196, 1975.

Chajek-Shaul T, Pisanty S, Knobler H, et al: HLA-B51 may serve as immunogenetic marker for a subgroup of patients with Behçet's syndrome. *Am J Med* 83: 666–671, 1987.

Clausen J, Bierring F: Fetal arterial involvement in Behçet's disease: An electron microscope study. *Acta Path Microbiol Immunol Scand Sect A* 91:133–136, 1983.

Cornelius F, Sigal-Nahum M, Gaulier A, et al: Behçet's disease with severe cutaneous necrotizing vasculitis: Response to plasma exchange. *J Am Acad Dermatol* 21:576–579, 1989.

Dietl S, Schumacher M, Menninger H, Lie JT: Subarachnoid hemorrhage associated with bilateral internal carotid artery aneurysms as a manifestation of Behçet's disease. *J Rheumatol* 21:775–776, 1994.

Dilsen N, Koniçe M, Aral O, et al: Behçet's disease associated with amyloidosis in Turkey and in the world. *Ann Rheum Dis* 47:157–163, 1988.

Dündar SV, Gençalp U, Şimşek H: Familial cases of Behçet's disease. *Br J Rheumatol* 113:319–321, 1985.

Dündar SV, Sivri B, Gököz A: Vasculitis of breast in Behçet's disease. *Angiology* 39:921–924, 1988.

Durieux P, Bletry O, Huchon G, et al: Multiple pulmonary arterial aneurysms in Behçet's disease and Hughes-Slovin syndrome. *Am J Med* 71:736–741, 1981.

Efthimiou J, Johnston C, Spiro SG, Turner-Warwick M: Pulmonary disease in Behçet's syndrome. *Q J Med* 58:259–280, 1986.

Emmi L, Salvati G, Brugnolo F, Marchione T: Immunopathological aspects of Behçet's disease. *Clin Exp Rheumatol* 13:687–691, 1995.

Fain O, Mathieu E, Lachassinne E, et al: Neonatal Behçet's disease. *Am J Med* 98:310–311, 1995.

Ferraz MB, Walter SD, Heymann R, Atra E: Sensitivity and specificity of different diagnostic criteria for Behçet's disease according to the latent class approach. *Br J Rheumatol* 34:932–935, 1995.

Gonzalez-Gay MA, Sanchez-Andrade A, Pulpeiro JR, et al: Hepatic arteritis in Behçet's disease. *J Rheumatol* 18:152–153, 1991.

Hamza M: Large artery involvement in Behçet's disease. *J Rheumatol* 14:554–559, 1987.

Herreman G, Beaufils H, Godeau P: Behçet's syndrome and renal involvement: A histological and immunofluorescent study of eleven patients. *Am J Med Sci* 284:10–17, 1982.

Hull RG, Harris EN, Gharavi AE, et al: Anticardiolipin antibodies: Occurrence in Behçet's syndrome. *Ann Rheum Dis* 43:746–748, 1984.

Hughes JP, Stovin PGI: Segmental pulmonary artery aneurysms with peripheral venous thrombosis. *Br J Dis Chest* 53:19–27, 1959.

Inaba G (ed): Behçet's Disease: Pathogenetic Mechanism and Clinical Feature. *Proceedings of the International Conference on Behçet's Disease, Tokyo, 1981.* Tokyo, University of Tokyo Press, 1982.

International Study Group for Behçet's Disease: Criteria for diagnosis of Behçet's disease. *Lancet* 335:1078–1080, 1990.

James DG, Spiteri MA: Behçet's disease. *Ophthalmology* 89:1279–1284, 1982.

James DG, Thomson A: Recognition of the diverse cardiovascular manifestations in Behçet's disease. *Am Heart J* 103:457–458, 1982.

Kaneko H, Nakajima H, Okamura A, et al: Histopathology of Behçet's disease. *Acta Pathol Jpn* 26:765–779, 197.

Kansu E, Özer FL, Akalin E, et al: Behçet's syndrome with obstruction of the venae cavae. *Q J Med* 41: 151–168, 1972.

Katoh K, Matsunaga K, Ishigatsubo Y, et al: Pathologically defined neuro-, vasculo-, entero-Behçet's disease. *J Rheumatol* 12:1186–1190, 1985.

Koç Y, Güllü I, Akpek G, et al: Vascular involvement in Behçet's disease. *J Rheumatol* 19:402–410, 1992.

Lakhanpal S, O'Duffy JD, Lie JT: Pathology. In Plotkin GR, Calabro JJ, O'Duffy JD (eds): *Behçet's Disease: A Contemporary Synopsis.* New York, Futura, 1989: 101–142.

Lakhanpal S, Tani K, Lie JT, et al: Pathologic features of Behçet's syndrome: A review of Japanese Autopsy Registry data. *Hum Pathol* 16:790–795, 1985.

Lang BA, Laxer RM, Thorner P, et al: Pediatric onset of Behçet's syndrome with myositis: Case report and literature review illustrating unusual features. *Arthritis Rheum* 33:418–425, 1990.

Lê Thi Huong D, Wechsler B, Papo T, et al: Arterial lesions in Behçet's disease: A study in 25 patients. *J Rheumatol* 22:2103–2113, 1995.

Lie JT: Cardiac and pulmonary manifestations of Behçet syndrome. *Path Res Pract* 183:347–352, 1988.

Lie JT: Vascular involvement in Behçet's disease: Arterial and venous and vessels of all sizes. *J Rheumatol* 19:341–343, 1992.

Mathur AK, Maslow J, Urffer PA: Hepatic arteritis in Behçet's disease. *J Rheumatol* 16:1516–1518, 1989.

Matsumoto T, Uekusa T, Fukuda Y: Vasculo-Behçet's disease; A pathologic study of eight cases. *Hum Pathol* 22:45–51, 1991.

O'Neill TW, Rigby AS, Silman AJ, Barnes C: Validation of the International Study Group criteria for Behçet's disease. *Br J Rheumatol* 33:115–117, 1994.

Özer ZG, Çetin M, Kahraman C: Thrombophlebitis in Behçet's disease. *VASA* 14:379–382, 1985.

Park JH, Han MC, Bettmann MA: Arterial manifestations of Behçet's disease. *Am J Roentgenol* 143:821–825, 1984.

Pereira R-M R, Gonçalves CR, Bueno C, et al: Anticardiolipin antibodies in Behçet's syndrome: A predictor of a more severe disease. *Clin Rheumatol* 8:289–291, 1989.

Plotkin GR, Calabro JJ, O'Duffy JD (eds): *Behçet's Disease: A Contemporary Synopsis.* New York, Futura, 1988, 314 pp.

Shimizu T, Ehrich GE, Inaba G, Hayashi K: Behçet's disease (Behçet's syndrome). *Semin Arthritis Rheum* 8: 223–260, 1977.

Slavin RE, de Groot WJ: Pathology of the lung in Behçet's disease: Case report and review of the literature. *Am J Surg Pathol* 5:779–788, 1981.

Tunaci A, Berkmen YM, Gökmen E: Thoracic involvement in Behçet's disease: Pathologic, clinical and imaging features. *Am J Roentgenol* 164:51–56, 1995.

Wolf SM, Schotland DL, Phillips LL: Involvement of nervous system in Behçet's syndrome. *Arch Neurol* 12:315–325, 1965.

Woodrow JC, Graham DR, Evans CC: Behçet's syndrome in HLA-identical siblings. *Br J Rheumatol* 29: 225–227, 1990.

Yazici H, Chamberlain MA, Tuzun Y, et al: A comparative study of the pathergy reaction among Turkish and British patients with Behçet's disease. *Ann Rheum Dis* 43:74–75, 1984.

Yurdakul S, Tüzüner N, Yurdakul I, et al: Amyloidosis in Behçet's syndrome. *Arthritis Rheum* 33:1586–1588, 1990.

Yurdakul S, Tüzüner N Yurdakul I, et al: Gastrointestinal involvement in Behçet's syndrome: A controlled study. *Ann Rheum Dis* 55:208–210, 1996.

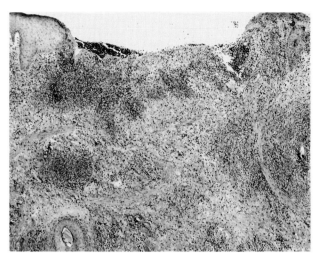

Figure 12.1. Aphthous ulcer in BD with eroded epidermis and an intense subepidermal mixed-cell inflammatory infiltrate.

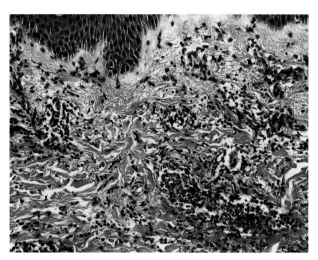

Figure 12.2. Cutaneous leukocytoclastic vasculitis in BD.

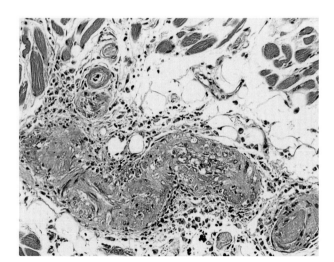

Figure 12.3. Polyarteritis-type small-vessel necrotizing vasculitis in a muscle biopsy of BD.

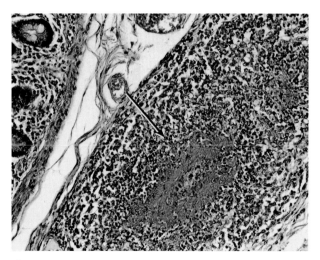

Figure 12.4. Submucosal necrotizing vasculitis (*arrow*) in a rectal biopsy of BD patient.

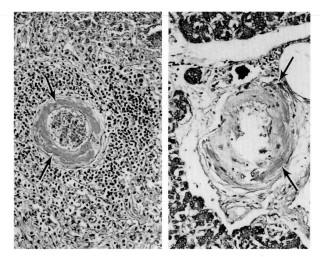

Figure 12.5. Vascular amyloidosis (*arrows*) in gastric (*left*) and pancreatic (*right*) biopsies.

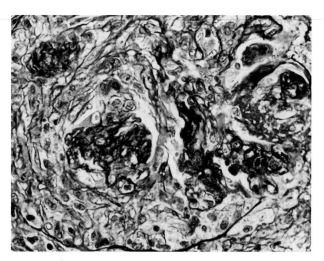

Figure 12.6. Focal necrotizing glomerulonephritis in a renal biopsy of BD patient.

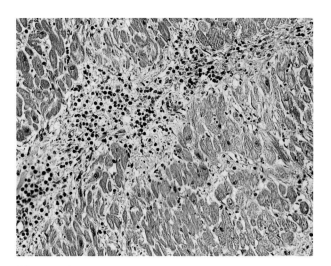

Figure 12.7. Lymphoplasmacytic myocarditis in BD patient with unexplained heart failure.

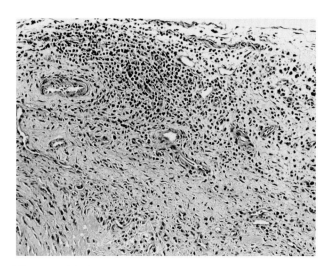

Figure 12.8. Lymphoplasmacytic aortic valvulitis in BD patient with aortic insufficiency.

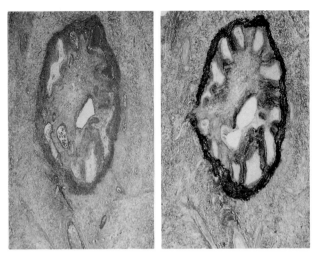

Figure 12.9. Matching H&E (*left*) and elastic stain (*right*) lung biopsy sections showing old, organized thrombus in BD patient with pulmonary thromboangiitis.

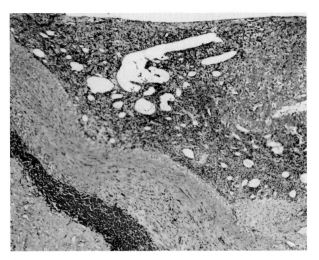

Figure 12.10. Organizing mural thrombus in an aneurysmal medium-sized pulmonary artery.

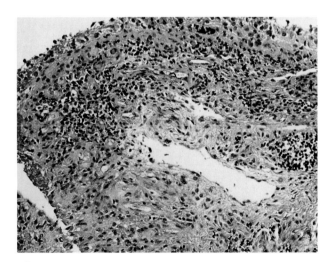

Figure 12.11. Knee joint synovitis with lymphoplasmacytic infiltrate and fibrin deposits in BD.

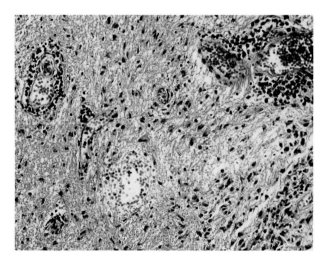

Figure 12.12. Brain biopsy in BD with lymphoplasmacytic infiltrate and small-vessel vasculitis.

13. Buerger's Disease

Buerger's disease is probably the least well understood and most tragic vascular occlusive disease of all time. It affects almost exclusively young male and female tobacco users during the most productive years of their life. When the disease is diagnosed early and if the patient abstains from tobacco, cure is virtually guaranteed without drug treatment, not even an aspirin; but when the diagnosis is missed or delayed, patients pay dearly with their legs and arms, or even with their life in extreme cases. Rheumatologists beware; the clinical presentation of Buerger's disease may mimic a connective tissue disorder with vasculitic complications, and corticosteroid treatment would have nothing to offer the patient except adverse drug side effects.

WHAT IS BUERGER'S DISEASE?

The earliest detailed description of Buerger's disease, or thromboangiitis obliterans (TAO), was provided by a little known young apprentice surgeon to the great Theodor Billroth of the Billroth gastrectomy fame, Felix von Winiwarter (1852–1931), in Vienna, in 1879. By sheer coincidence, that happened to be the year and place of birth of Dr. Leo Buerger (1879–1943), the American surgeon who published the first English-language account of the disease, later named after him, 29 years later, when he was working at the Mount Sinai Hospital in New York.

Buerger's disease, known in Europe as *Morbus Winiwarter-Buerger,* is a nonatherosclerotic, segmental, and usually recurrent and progressive inflammatory vaso-occlusive disease of unknown etiology. A proposed pathogenetic mechanism for Buerger's disease involves the interaction between the coagulation system, its control proteins (antithrombin III, protein C, and protein S) and the endothelium (Fig. 13.1). Clinical experience clearly indicates Buerger's disease is closely tied to the active and, rarely, passive exposure to tobacco smoking, with onset of symptoms and signs of the disease usually before the age of 40, and may be as early as 14 years; and males are affected almost ten times more commonly than are females. Most but not all of the patients are heavy smokers. The susceptible persons may be exquisitely sensitive to tobacco use; once affected, smoking even one cigarette can trigger the reappearance of symptoms and signs of the disease after a "remission" from total abstinence of tobacco use.

BUERGER'S DISEASE IN WOMEN

Buerger's disease in women is uncommon and the reported incidence was only 1 to 2% in most published series of cases before 1970. Several more recently published series, however, showed an almost tenfold increase of Buerger's disease in women: 22.6% in a Swiss study (Leu 1985); 11% in the Rochester, Minnesota, study (Lie 1987); 19% in the Portland, Oregon, study (Mills et al. 1987); 14% in the Yugoslavia study (Pirnat and Simic 1988); and 23% in the Cleveland, Ohio, study (Olin et al. 1990). It is unclear whether the greater number of smokers among young women in recent decades and, perhaps the effect of passive smoking on susceptible persons, are responsible for the marked increase of Buerger's disease in women. Of interest, the incidence of Buerger's disease among Japanese women still remains relatively low and fairly constant.

CLINICAL RECOGNITION OF BUERGER'S DISEASE

Buerger's disease is uncommon but not rare. The disease has a worldwide distribution, being more prevalent in the Orient, Southeast Asia, India, Middle East, and Eastern Europe. Imprecise and ill-conceived clinical and pathologic criteria are largely responsible for the widespread and continued uncertainty and confusion in the diagnosis and management of Buerger's disease.

The clinical diagnostic criteria for Buerger's disease, as proposed by Shionoya in 1990 are: (1) tobacco smoking history; (2) onset of disease before 40 years of age; (3) infrapopliteal vaso-occlusive lesions; (4) either upper limb involvement or migrating thrombophlebitis; and (5) absence of atherosclerosis risk factors other than smoking. A diagnosis of Buerger's disease can be made when all five criteria are met, preferably also with supportive arteriographic findings.

According to Papa and Adar (1992), apart from the three *basic* observations emphasized by Leo Buerger—young age, male gender, and tobacco use—one needs to consider three *additional* essential clinical criteria for the diagnosis of TAO: upper limb involvement, superficial thrombophlebitis, and vasospastic (Raynaud's) phenomenon. At least two of three *additional* features are required for a "definite" diagnosis of TAO; and one or none for "probable" or "suspected" category, respectively. Thus, the criteria for the diagnosis of Buerger's disease as proposed by Papa and Adar (1992) for Israeli patients, are virtually identical to those by Shionoya (1990) for Japanese patients.

ARTERIOGRAPHIC FINDINGS

Angiographically, multiple segmental occlusions of the distal arteries in the lower or upper limbs are characteristic of Buerger's disease, with each occlusion being abrupt or tapered. The arterial lumen proximal to the occlusion is usually smooth and regular. A corrugated or accordion-like appearance is sometimes observed, mostly in the femoral or crural arteries, which may represent vasospasm. There is usually an extensive network of collateral vessels around each occlusion so that circulation distal to the obstruction may be maintained, at least initially; these collateral vessels have a "corkscrew" or "tree root-like" configuration (Fig. 13.2). Unlike arteriosclerosis obliterans, neither calcification in the vessel wall nor a "moth-eaten" defect of the arterial-lumen silhouette is seen angiographically in Buerger's disease.

BIOPSY DIAGNOSIS OF BUERGER'S DISEASE

TAO is an intriguing vaso-occlusive disease. It affects principally the medium-sized and small arteries *and veins* of the lower and upper limbs, and only rarely of the viscera. There is virtually no known involvement of the aorta, venae cavae, or pulmonary and cerebral blood vessels, with acceptable biopsy documentation of the disease.

Buerger's disease is fundamentally an *inflammatory thrombosis affecting both arteries and veins,* and the histopathology of the affected blood vessels varies according to the chronologic age of the disease when the vascular lesions are biopsied. The histopathology is most likely to be diagnostic at the early phase of the disease, especially veins with acute thrombophlebitis. The histopathology evolves to changes in arteries and veins considered to be consistent with or suggestive of subacute phase or intermediate stage of the disease, and becomes virtually indeterminate or nondiagnostic at end-stage or chronic phase, say, in an amputated limb, when all that remain are gangrene and old organized

thrombi with dense fibrous scarring of the affected arteries and veins.

Acute Phase Lesions

The early or acute phase vascular lesions of Buerger's disease are characterized by an intense inflammation of the vessel wall associated with occlusive thrombosis, most evident in the affected veins and the inflammation may precede the thrombosis (Fig. 13.3). Around the periphery of the occlusive thrombus, there are frequently one or more small clusters of polymorphonuclear leukocytes with karyorrhexis, the so-called "microabscesses," in which one or more multinucleated giant cells may be present (Fig. 13.4) and sometimes a true "granuloma" coexists with the microabscess (Fig. 13.5). This histologic finding, while not pathognomonic, is almost diagnostic of Buerger's disease; it has been observed by the author in only two other conditions, namely, the thrombophlebitis in Behçet's disease and in Wegener's granulomatosis. The same finding occurs infrequently in the arteries, where it may persist to the stage of early organization of the occlusive thrombus (Fig. 13.6).

Subacute Phase and End-Stage Lesions

Progressive organization of the occlusive thrombus in the artery and vein signifies the subacute phase lesion, and the thrombus organization is usually accompanied by a prominent inflammatory cell infiltrate in Buerger's disease (Fig. 13.7). The end-stage lesion is characterized by completed organization of the occlusive thrombus with rather prominent neoangiogenesis (vascularization) and recanalization of the thrombus and adventitial fibrosis (Fig. 13.8). Throughout all phases of Buerger's disease (acute, subacute, and chronic), the normal vessel architecture including the internal elastic lamina remains essentially intact and this feature distinguishes TAO from arteriosclerosis obliterans and from systemic vasculitides, in which there is usually more striking disruption of the internal elastic lamina and media.

VASCULAR LESIONS IN UNUSUAL SITUATIONS

Leo Buerger, in his 1924 monograph on TAO was the first to describe the possible involvement of mesenteric vessels in four patients. To date, there are fewer than 20 reported cases of Buerger's disease with biopsy proven digestive tract involvement (Fig. 13.9), about equally divided between small and large intestines. In the same monograph, Buerger described the occasional involvement of testicular and spermatic cord arteries and veins, which is even more rare (Fig. 13.10). There has been no more than a handful of known cases of Buerger's disease involving the superficial temporal artery of young smokers (Fig. 13.11), in some the temporal artery lesions had been preceded by peripheral limb ischemia requiring amputation. Verging on being truly a pathologic curiosity was a unique case of Buerger's disease in a saphenous vein coronary artery bypass graft (Fig. 13.12).

BIBLIOGRAPHY

Adar R, Papa MZ, Halpern Z, et al: Cellular sensitivity to collagen in thromboangiitis obliterans. *N Engl J Med* 308:1113–1116, 1983.

Biller J, Asconagé J Challa VR, et al: A case for cerebral thromboangiitis obliterans. *Stroke* 12:686–689, 1981.

Broide E, Scapa E, Peer A, et al: Buerger's disease presenting as acute small bowel ischemia. *Gastroenterology* 104:1192–1195, 1993.

Buerger L: Thromboangiitis obliterans: A study of the vascular lesions leading to presenile spontaneous gangrene. *Am J Med Sci* 136:567–580, 1908.

Buerger L: *The Circulatory Disturbances of the Extremities Including Gangrene, Vasomotor, and Trophic Changes.* Philadelphia, W B Saunders, 1924.

Cebezas-Moya R, Dragstedt LR II: An extreme example of Buerger's disease. *Arch Surg* 101:632–634, 1971.

Dible JH: *The Pathology of the Limb Ischaemia.* Edinburgh, Oliver & Boyd, 1966:79–86.

Fisher CM: Cerebral thromboangiitis obliterans: Including a critical review of the literature. *Medicine* 36:169–209, 1957.

Gilkes R, Dow J: Aortic involvement in Buerger's disease. *Br J Radiol* 46:110–114, 1973.

Gores I, Burrows S: A reconsideration of the pathogenesis of Buerger's disease. *Am J Clin Pathol* 29:319–330, 1958.

Gulati SM, Madhra K, Thusoo TK, et al: Autoantibodies in thromboangiitis obliterans (Buerger's disease). *Angiology* 33:642–651, 1982.

Goodman RM, Elian B, Mozes M, Deutsch V: Buerger's disease in Israel. *Am J Med* 39:601–615, 1965.

Harkavy J: Tobacco sensitiveness in thromboangiitis obliterans, migratory phlebitis, and coronary artery disease. *Bull N Y Acad Sci* 9:318–322, 1933.

Horwitz O: Buerger's disease revisited. *Ann Intern Med* 55:341–344, 1961.

Inada K, Katsumura T: The entity of Buerger's disease. *Angiology* 23:668–687, 1972.

Kinare SG, Kher YR, Rao G, et al: Patterns of occlusive peripheral vascular disease in India. *Angiology* 27:165–180, 1976.

Lambeth JT, Yong NK: Arteriographic findings in thromboangiitis obliterans: With emphasis on femoro-popliteal involvement. *Am J Roentgenol* 109:553–562, 1970.

Lie JT: Thromboangiitis obliterans (Buerger's disease) in women. *Medicine* 64:65–72, 1987.

Lie JT: Thromboangiitis (Buerger's disease) in a saphenous vein arterial graft. *Hum Pathol* 18:402–404, 1987.

Lie JT: Thromboangiitis obliterans (Buerger's disease) in an elderly man after cessation of cigarette smoking—A case report. *Angiology* 38:864–867, 1987.

Lie JT: Thromboangiitis obliterans (Buerger's disease) revisited. *Pathol Annu* 23(2): 257–291, 1988.

Lie JT: Thromboangiitis obliterans (Buerger's disease) and smokeless tobacco. Arthritis Rheum 31:812–813, 1988.

Lie JT: The rise and fall and resurgence of thromboangiitis obliterans (Buerger's disease). *Acta Pathol Jpn* 39:153–158, 1989.

Lie JT, Mann RJ, Ludwig J: The brothers von Winiwarter, Alexander (1848–1917) and Felix (1852–1931), and thromboangiitis obliterans. *Mayo Clin Proc* 54:802–807, 1979.

Lie JT, Michet CJ, Jr: Thromboangiitis obliterans with eosinophilia (Buerger's disease) of the temporal arteries. *Hum Pathol* 19:598–602, 1988.

Mavor GE: Thromboangiitis obliterans: Clinical and angiographic findings with discussion on clinical diagnosis. *Q J Med* 24:229–244, 1955.

McKusick VA, Harris WS: The Buerger syndrome in the Orient. *Bull Johns Hopkins Hosp* 109:241–291, 1961.

McKusick VA, Harris WS, et al: Buerger's disease: A distinct clinical and pathologic entity. *JAMA* 181:5–12, 1962.

Nielobowicz J, Rosnowski A, Pruszynski B, et al: Nat-

146 MISCELLANEOUS RELATED DISORDERS

ural history of Buerger's disease. *J Cardiovasc Surg* 21:529–540, 1980.

Olin JW, Lie JT: Thromboangiitis obliterans (Buerger's disease). In Loscalzo J, Creager MA, Dzou (eds): *Vascular Medicine,* ed 2. Boston, Little, Brown and Co, 1996:1033–1049.

Olin JW, Young JR, Graor RA, et al: The changing clinical spectrum of thromboangiitis obliterans (Buerger's disease). *Circulation* 82 (suppl IV): 3–8, 1990.

Papa MZ, Adar R: A critical look at thromboangiitis obliterans (Buerger's disease). *Persp Vasc Surg* 5: 1–21, 1992.

Shionoya S: *Buerger's Disease: Pathology, Diagnosis*

and Treatment. Nagoya, The University of Nagoya Press, 1990, 261 pp.

Shionoya S, Leu HJ, Lie JT: Buerger's disease (thromboangiitis obliterans). In Stehbens WE, Lie JT (eds): *Vascular Pathology.* London, Chapman & Hall, 1995: 657–678.

Vink M (ed): Symposium on Buerger's disease. *J Cardiovasc Surg* 14:1–51, 1973.

Wessler S: Buerger's disease revisited. *Surg Clin North Am* 49:703–713, 1969.

Williams G: Recent view on Buerger's disease. *J Clin Pathol* 22:573–578, 1969.

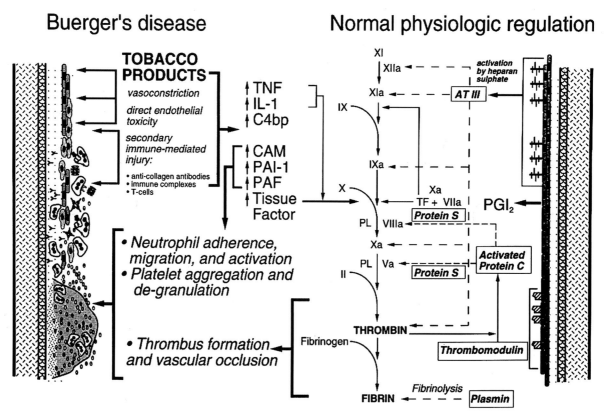

Figure 13.1. Current hypothesis of the pathogenesis of thrombosis in Buerger's disease. The interactions between the coagulation system, its control proteins, and the endothelium are illustrated schematically. *Abbreviations:* AT III=antithrombin III; CAM=cellular adhesion molecule; C4bp=C4 binding protein; IL-1= interlukin 1; PAF=platelet activating factor; PAI-1=plasminogen activator inhibitor; PGI$_2$=prostacyclin; TNF=tumor necrosis factor. *(Courtesy of Dr. Kevin Davies)*

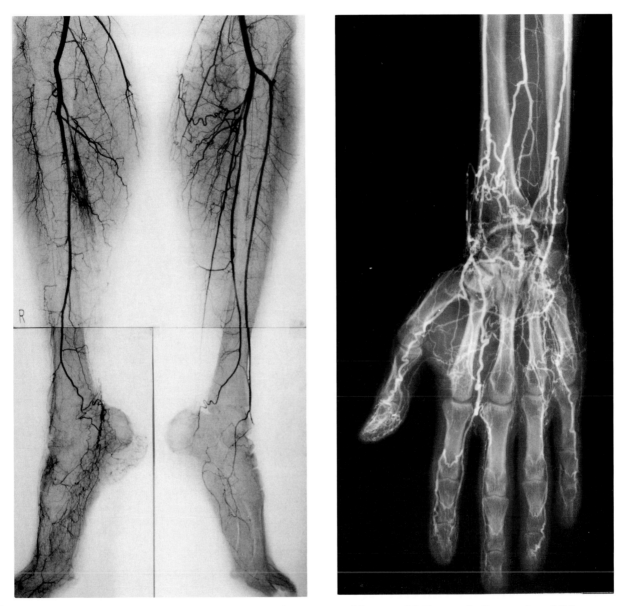

Figure 13.2. Left. Bilateral femoral arteriogram of a 31-year-old man with Buerger's disease. In addition to multiple small-vessel occlusions in the feet and toes, the right anterior and posterior tibial arteries are occluded near their origins; the left posterior tibial artery shows tapering occlusion and the anterior tibial artery ends abruptly at the ankle. **Right.** Right brachial arteriogram of one 46-year-old man with Buerger's disease, showing multiple occlusions of arteries of the forearm, hand and fingers, and collaterals. *(Courtesy of Prof. Shigehiko Shionoya)*

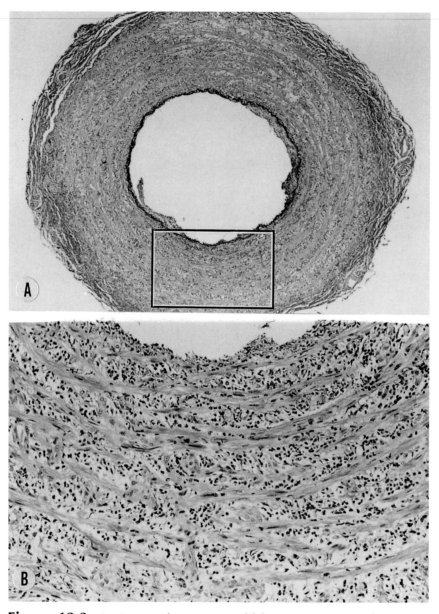

Figure 13.3. A. Acute subcutaneous phlebitis in Buerger's disease. **B.** Close-up view of the boxed area in **A** to show an intense mixed-cell inflammatory infiltrate in the venous vessel wall. *With permission from Lie JT. Pathol Annu* 1988;23(2):257–291.

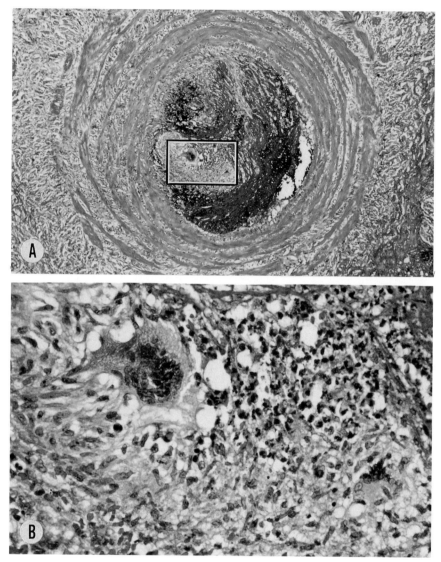

Figure 13.4. **A.** Typical acute phase lesion of Buerger's disease in a sub-cutaneous vein with thrombophlebitis. **B.** Close-up view of the boxed lesion in **A** to show multinucleated giant cells in an intraluminal microabscess. *With permission from Lie JT. Pathol Annu* 1988;23(2):257–291.

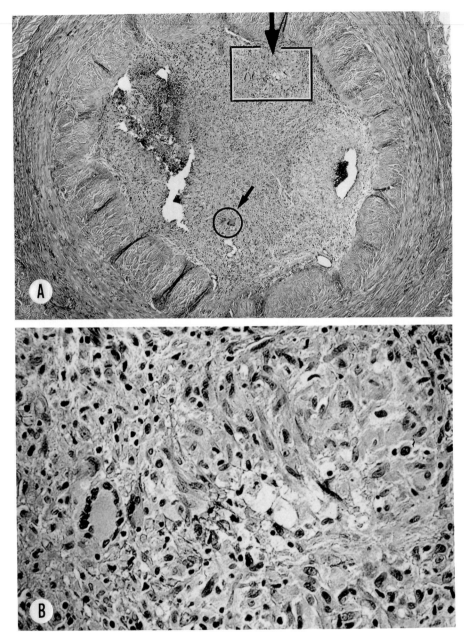

Figure 13.5. A. Thrombophlebitis in acute phase Buerger's disease with microabscesses and granulomatous inflammation (*rectangle*) and giant cells (*circle*). **B.** Close-up view of rectangle in **A** to show the giant cells.

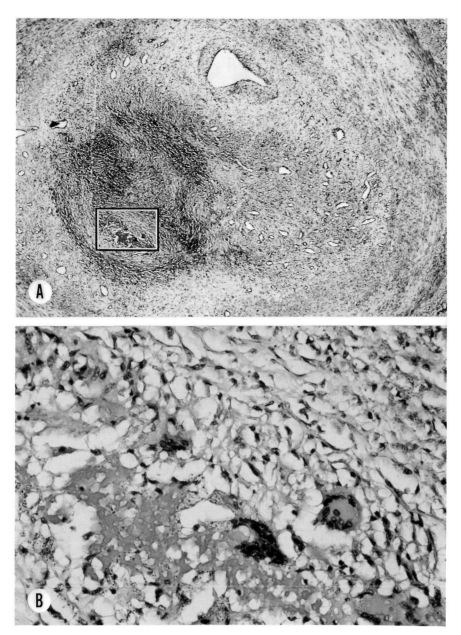

Figure 13.6. **A.** Occluded femoral artery in Buerger's disease with a resolving microabscess in the organized thrombus (*rectangle*). **B.** Close-up view of several giant cells in the microabscess.

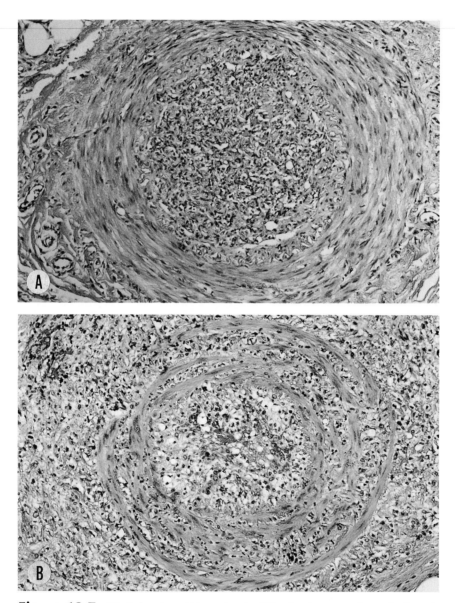

Figure 13.7. Digital artery **(A)** and vein **(B)** of subacute phase lesions in Buerger's disease showing early organization of occlusive thrombi with prominent neoangiogenesis and inflammatory reaction. *With permission from Lie JT. Pathol Annu* 1988;23(2):257–291.

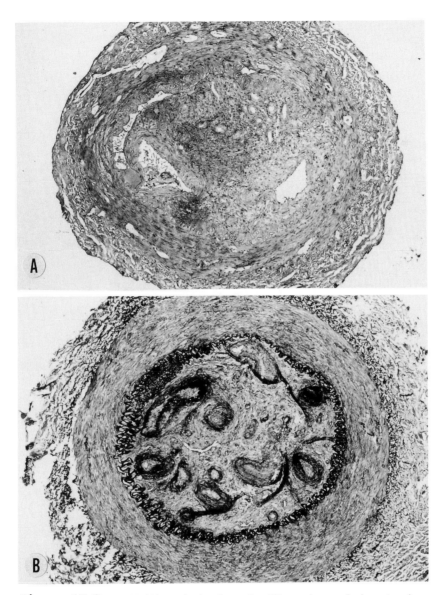

Figure 13.8. H&E **(A)** and elastic stain **(B)** sections of chronic phase arterial lesion in Buerger's disease showing recanalization of organized thrombus with essentially intact internal elastic lamina. *With permission from Lie JT. Pathol Annu* 1988;23(2):257–291.

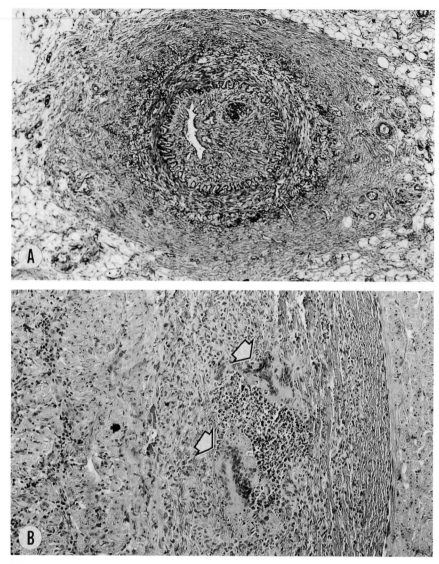

Figure 13.9. Mesenteric vascular lesions of artery **(A)** with organizing thrombus, and vein **(B)** with giant cells in microabscess of thrombus (*arrows*) in Buerger's disease. *With permission from Lie JT. Pathol Annu* 1988; 23(2):257–291.

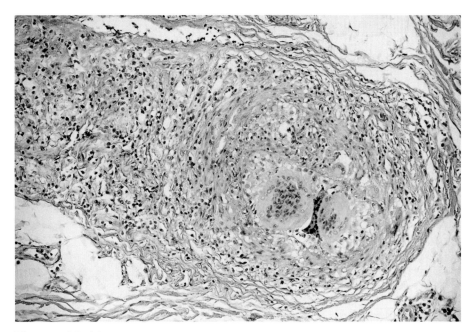

Figure 13.10. Testicular vein acute phase lesion of Buerger's disease with granulomatous inflammation and giant cells in the thrombus.

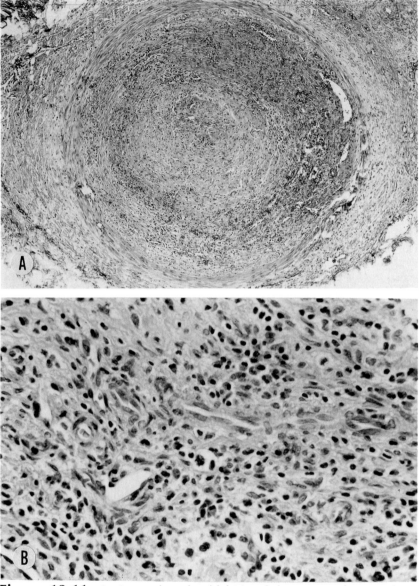

Figure 13.11. **A.** Acute thrombophlebitis of the temporal artery in a patient with Buerger's disease. **B.** Close-up view of the inflammatory infiltrate with prominent eosinophils. *With permission from Lie JT. Pathol Annu 1988;23(2):257–291.*

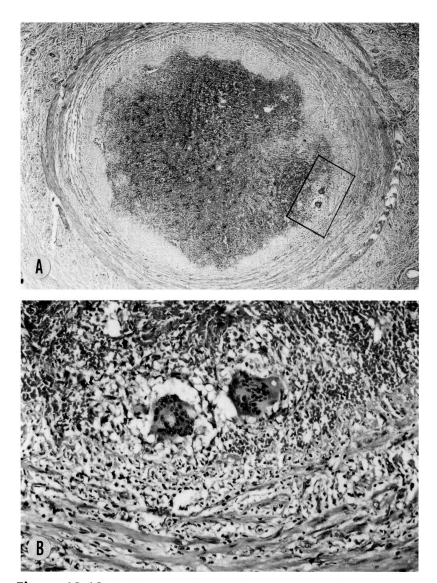

Figure 13.12. A. Buerger's disease of coronary artery bypass saphenous vein graft. **B.** Close-up view of the boxed area in **A** to show the microabscess and giant cells in the occlusive thrombus. *With permission from Lie JT. Pathol Annu* 1988;23(2):257–291.

14. Cogan Syndrome

In 1945, Dr. David Cogan of the Massachusetts Eye and Ear Infimary, Boston, first described a new clinical syndrome of nonsyphilitic interstitial keratitis and audiovestibular symptoms; and fifteen years later, Dr. Thane Cody of the Mayo Clinic, Rochester, Minnesota, was the first to emphasize the systemic manifestations of this syndrome. Cogan syndrome is to be differentiated from *Cogan's oculomotor apraxia, Cogan's corneal dystrophy,* and the *Cogan-Reese iris-naevus syndrome.*

Cogan syndrome is an uncommon disease of young adults and older children, of equal gender distribution, with probably fewer than 100 cases having been reported in the English-language literature. Vestibuloauditory symptoms are acute in onset, usually precede the ocular disorder, and may be confused with Menière's disease. About 50% of patients also have one or more systemic manifestations that include systemic vasculitis, aortitis and aortic valvular disease, myocarditis, lymphadenopathy, gastrointestinal hemorrhage, renal parenchymal disease, and musculoskeletal disorders. Thus, the rheumatologists and physicians of other subspecialties may be called upon to diagnose and manage patients with Cogan syndrome.

The etiology of Cogan syndrome is unknown. A temporal association has been noted with smallpox vaccination or upper respiratory tract infection, but investigators have failed to confirm theories for an infective etiology, including the incrimination of *Chlamydia psittaci, Chlamydia trachomatis,* and *Borrelia burgdorferi* microorganisms. Initial reports of the association with HLA-BW17 antigen remain unsubstantiated; there is limited evidence of autoimmune reactivity to both corneal and inner-ear antigens; and the presence of lymphocytes in vestibulo-auditory and ocular tissue that may represent cell-mediated changes has not been consistently observed in all the biopsy specimens procured.

The most common abnormal laboratory test in Cogan syndrome is a moderate elevation of the erythrocyte sedimentation rate, and patients may also have mild to moderate anemia, leukocytosis, and thrombocytosis. In symptomatic patients, angiographic studies often may demonstrate abnormalities suggestive of visceral vasculitis, aortitis, and/or aortic insufficiency.

The diagnosis of Cogan syndrome is essentially established on a careful clinico-angiographic evaluation of the patient. Biopsy plays a limited role and, as always, it requires clinicopathologic correlations in all suspected cases, because there are no pathognomonic histopathologic changes.

The pertinent biopsy findings, where tissue samples are available for examination, may include a lymphoplasmacytic aortic valvulitis (Fig. 14.1) and/or aortitis (Fig. 14.2); nonspecific myocarditis (Fig. 14.3); cutaneous leukocytoclastic vasculitis (Fig. 14.4); intestinal necrotizing vasculitis (Fig. 14.5); and combined tubulointerstitial-focal segmental necrotizing glomerulonephritis (Fig. 14.6).

BIBLIOGRAPHY

Bicknell JM, Holland JV: Neurologic manifestations of Cogan syndrome. *Neurology* 28:278–281, 1978.

Bielory L, Conti J, Frohman L: Immunologic grand rounds: Cogan's syndrome. *J Allergy Clin Immunol* 85:808–815, 1990.

Cheson BD, Bluming AZ, Alroy J: Cogan's syndrome: A systemic vasculitis. *Am J Med* 60:549–555, 1976.

Cody DTR, Williams HL: Cogan's syndrome. *Laryngoscope* 70:477–478, 1960.

Cody DTR, Williams HL: Cogan's syndrome. *Mayo Clin Proc* 37:372–375, 1962.

Cogan DG: Syndrome of nonsyphilitic interstitial keratitis and vestibuloauditory symptoms. *Arch Ophthalmol* 33:144–149, 1945.

Cogan DG, Dickersin GR: Nonsyphilitic interstitial keratitis with vestibuloauditory symptoms: A case with fatal aortitis. *Arch Ophthalmol* 71:172–175, 1962.

Del Carpio J, Espinosa LR, Osterland CK: Cogan's syndrome and HLA BW17 (letter to the editor). *N Engl J Med* 295:1262–1263, 1976.

Editorial: Cogan's syndrome. *Lancet* 337:1011–1012, 1991.

Edstrom S, Vahlne A: Immunological findings in a case of Cogan's syndrome. *Acta Otolaryngol* 82:212–215, 1976.

Eisenstein B, Taubenhaus M: Nonsyphilitic interstitial keratitis and bilateral deafness (Cogan's syndrome) associated with cardiovascular disease. *N Engl J Med* 258:1074–1079, 1958.

Fisher ER, Hellstrom HR: Cogan's syndrome and systemic vascular disease: Analysis of pathologic features. *Arch Pathol* 72:572–592, 1961.

Gelfand ML, Kantor T, Gorstein F: Cogan's syndrome with cardiovascular involvement: Aortic insufficiency. *Bull NY Acad Sci* 48:647–660, 1972.

Gilbert WS, Talbot FJ: Cogan's syndrome: Signs of peri-arteritis nodosa and cerebral venous thrombosis. *Arch Ophthalmol* 82:633–636, 1969.

Haynes BF, Kaiser-Kupfer MI, Mason P, Fauci AS: Cogan syndrome: Studies in thirteen patients, long-term follow-up, and a review of the literature. *Medicine* 59:426–441, 1980.

Hughes GB, Kinney SE, Barna B, et al: Autoimmune reactivity in Cogan's syndrome: A preliminary report. *Otolaryngol Head Neck Surg* 91:24–32, 1983.

Kaiser-Kupfer MI, Mittal KK, Del Valle LA, et al: The HLA antigens in Cogan's syndrome. *Am J Ophthalmol* 86:314–316, 1978.

LaRaja RD: Cogan syndrome associated with mesenteric vascular insufficiency. *Arch Surg* 111:1028–1031, 1976.

Oliner L, Taubenhaus M, Shapira TM, Leshin N: Non-syphilitic interstitial keratitis and bilateral deafness (Cogan's syndrome) associated with essential polyangitis (periarteritis nodosa): A review of the syndrome with consideration of a possible pathogenic mechanism. *N Engl J Med* 248:1001–1008, 1953.

Pinals RS: Cogan's syndrome with arthritis and aortic insufficiency. *J Rheumatol* 5:294–298, 1978.

Vollertsen RS: Vasculitis and Cogan's syndrome. *Rheum Dis Clin N Am* 16:433–439, 1990.

Vollertsen RS, McDonald TJ, Younge BR, et al: Cogan's syndrome: 18 cases and a review of the literature. *Mayo Clin Proc* 61:344–361, 1986.

Wilder-Smith E, Roelcke U: Cogan's syndrome. *J Clin Neuro-Ophthalmol* 10:261–263, 1990.

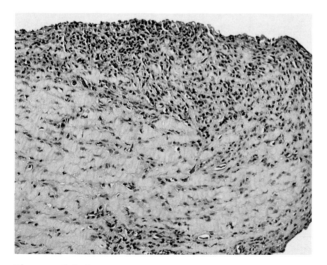

Figure 14.1. Lymphoplasmacytic aortic valvulitis in Cogan syndrome with symptomatic aortic insufficiency requiring surgical intervention.

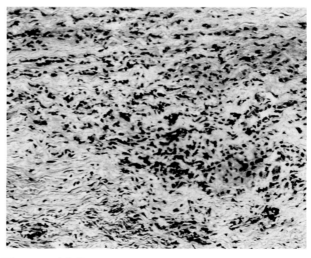

Figure 14.2. Lymphoplasmacytic aortitis in Cogan syndrome with aortic insufficiency.

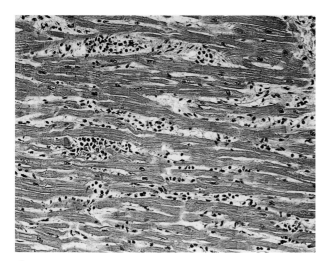

Figure 14.3. Biopsy finding of nonspecific myocarditis in Cogan syndrome with unexplained heart failure.

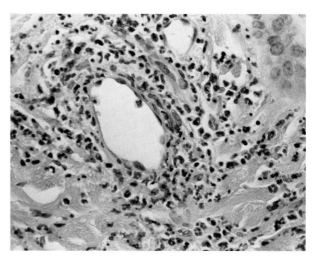

Figure 14.4. Cutaneous leukocytoclastic vasculitis in Cogan syndrome with skin petechiae.

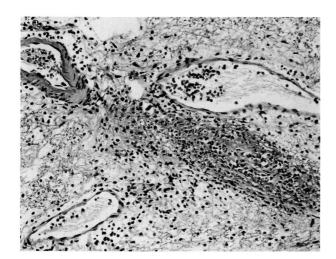

Figure 14.5. Necrotizing vasculitis in small bowel biopsy of a Cogan syndrome patient with gastrointestinal hemorrhage.

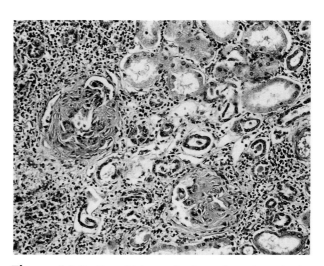

Figure 14.6. Renal biopsy finding of combined tubulointerstitial-focal segmental necrotizing glomerulonephritis in Cogan syndrome.

15. Eosinophilic Fasciitis, Eosinophilia-Myalgia and Toxic-Oil Syndromes

EOSINOPHILIC FASCIITIS

In 1974, Lawrence Shulman described two patients with scleroderma-like skin changes, which he designated as "diffuse fasciitis with hypergammaglobulinemia and eosinophilia." In 1975, Gerald Rodnan et al. independently reported six patients with the same scleroderma-like syndrome, which they called "eosinophilic fasciitis." Subsequently, it becomes apparent that the peripheral blood and tissue eosinophilia may be variable and, hence, the term "diffuse fasciitis with or without eosinophilia" was used in the proposed American Rheumatism Association 1983 nomenclature and classification of arthritis and rheumatism. The cause of eosinophilic fasciitis remains unknown; only in the past decade has its occurrence after allogeneic bone marrow transplantation and after the ingestion of L-tryptophan been documented in the literature.

Eosinophilic fasciitis is relatively uncommon but not rare; in the first 15 years since its 1974 original description over 200 cases (including 18 children and 2 adult siblings) have been reported in the English-language literature. All of the patients share the same clinical characteristics of a scleroderma-like disease without Raynaud's phenomenon and, in many cases, exercise has been cited as a precipitating event. The major clinical manifestation is usually symmetric inflammatory swelling and induration of the arms and legs, with infrequent involvement of the trunk and often sparing of the hands and feet. Visceral involvement is often mild and asymptomatic, but the association with hematologic disorders, such as hypergammaglobulinemia, aplastic anemia, and thrombocytopenia, carries a poorer prognosis.

The diagnostic confirmation of eosinophilic fasciitis requires a full-thickness *en bloc* incisional biopsy that includes the skin, subcutaneous fat, fascia, and superficial muscle in continuity. Inflammation, edema, and sclerotic thickening of the fascia are histopathologic hallmarks of eosinophilic fasciitis. Early in the course of the disease, the lower subcutis and deep fascia are infiltrated with lymphocytes, plasma cells, histiocytes, and eosinophils (Fig. 15.1). Distribution of the eosinophils may be focal and there appears to be a close correlation between peripheral blood and tissue eosinophilia (Fig. 15.2). As the disease progresses, the subcutis, fascia, and eventually the dermis become collagenized, thick-

ened, and sclerotic, corresponding to the well-known tightly bound with irregular dimpling of the skin over the affected areas. An eosinophilic myositis may occur in association with or independently of eosinophilic fasciitis. True vasculitis in eosinophilic fasciitis is rare.

EOSINOPHILIA-MYALGIA AND TOXIC-OIL SYNDROMES

Eosinophilia-myalgia syndrome (EMS) and toxic-oil syndrome (TOS) are unique food/drug/toxin induced systemic diseases that share clinical and pathologic manifestations with scleroderma and eosinophilic fasciitis. EMS was first recognized in the United States, in October 1989, as a new disease associated with L-tryptophan ingestion; a short-lived epidemic soon followed with about 2000 patients identified some 12 months later, but additional cases seemingly declined just as abruptly after withdrawal of L-tryptophan from the market. The development of EMS in the United States drew attention to and comparison with the previously described epidemic of TOS in Spain, during 1981 and the ensuing 18 months, affecting people after ingestion of adulterated rapeseed oil. The remarkable clinical and pathologic overlaps of EMS and TOS (Table 15.1), their rise and fall corresponding to the introduction and elimination of the offending toxins, respectively, highlight the important role of epidemiologic investigations in identifying and incriminating environmental hazards and culprits as the cause of autoimmune diseases.

The Centers for Disease Control define EMS as (1) peripheral blood eosinophil count >1000 cells/mm^3, (2) myalgia severe enough to limit usual daily activities, and (3) no evidence of infection or neoplasm that could explain the first two criteria.

Mucocutaneous Manifestations

The principal mucocutaneous manifestation is the development of skin thickening and changes that resemble the findings in scleroderma and eosinophilic fasciitis (Figs. 15.1 and 15.2). These skin changes begin in the initial 3 to 6 months of the disease and are often associated with cutaneous papular mucinosis; their distribution may be diffuse, limited or localized, and may be associated with hyperpigmentation.

Table 15.1 Comparison of the Eosinophilia-Myalgia Syndrome (EMS) and Toxic-Oil Syndrome (TOS)

	EMS	TOS
Historical Data		
First notification	October 1989	May 1981
End of epidemic	December 1990	December 1982
Percent of women affected	84	67
Average age of patients (yr)	49	34
Peak number of reported cases	2,000 in 2 years	20,000 in 3 years
Mortality	36 deaths (1 in 55)	351 deaths (1 in 57)
Toxin identified	Contaminant in L-tryptophan	Adulterated rapeseed oil
Clinicopathologic Features		
Generalized myalgia	+++	++
Fasciitis	++	++
Scleroderma-like skin	+	+
Skin rash	++	++
Arthralgia/arthritis	+	+
Peripheral neuropathy	++	++
Pulmonary involvement	++	++
Cardiac involvement	+	+
CNS involvement	±	±
Laboratory Findings		
Peripheral blood eosinophilia	+++	++
Anemia	+	+
Thrombocytopenia or thrombocytosis	+	+
Elevated IgE	±	±
Immune complexes	Not detected	Not detected
ANA (speckled pattern)	+	+
Tissue eosinophilia	+++	++
Lymphocytic infiltrate	+++	+++
Small-vessel vasculitis/microangiopathy	+	++
Thromboembolism	+	++

Neuromuscular and Vascular Manifestations

The acute onset of incapacitating myalgia is one of the principal hallmarks of EMS, and myalgia may persist, although less incapacitating, in 50 to 90% of patients at up to 3 years of follow-up. The myopathic changes in biopsies are predominantly perimyositis with variable degrees of eosinophilic infiltrate (Fig. 15.3), small-vessel perivascular infiltrates (Fig. 15.4) and, only rarely, a true vasculitis. Severe hyperesthesia and paresthesia that accompany the acute myalgia signal the development of peripheral neuropathy, often with an ascending component mimicking Guillain-Barré syndrome. Depending on the procurement time in relation to the symptomatic age of the disease, a peripheral biopsy may show small-vessel vasculitis (Fig. 15. 5) in the acute stage or axonal degeneration and atrophy in the chronic stage. A rare case of eosinophilic non-giant cell temporal arteritis (Fig. 15.6) was the unexpected biopsy finding in a 57-year-old woman who had a new onset headache as one of the presenting symptoms of EMS.

Cardiopulmonary Manifestations

Cardiac involvement was cited to occur in approximately 9% of 210 patients with EMS in a large national survey with 18 to 24-month follow-up. Clinically documented abnormalities include sinus tachycardia, myocarditis, coronary artery vasospasm, and right ventricular dysfunction secondary to pulmonary hypertension. Endomyocardial biopsies in EMS patients presenting with unexplained heart failure may show an eosinophilic myocarditis (Figs. 15.7 and 15.8) and, much more infrequently, endomyocardial fibrosis.

Autopsy studies of the heart in patients succumbing to EMS have revealed small-vessel proliferative vasculopathy and ganglioneuritis.

Clinically, dyspnea and/or cough accompanied by pulmonary interstitial or alveolar infiltrates and/or pleural effusions occur in 15 to 50% of EMS patients. In most large series and long-term follow-up studies, respiratory symptoms continued to be present in similar proportions of cases. Open-lung biopsies in acute cases have revealed hypersensitivity pneumonitis with eosinophilic infiltrate (Fig. 15.9) and, less commonly, bronchiolitis obliterans (Fig. 15.10) and a small-vessel pulmonary vasculitis (Fig. 15.11). A proliferative occlusive vascular disease with pulmonary hypertension (Fig. 15.12) have been observed in both EMS and TOS, especially in later stage of the disease and in longer-term follow-up of patients.

BIBLIOGRAPHY

Alonso-Ruiz A, Zea-Mendoza AC, Salazar-Vallinas JM, et al: Toxic oil syndrome: A syndrome with features overlapping those of various forms of scleroderma. *Semin Arthritis Rheum* 15:200–212, 1986.

Barnes L, Rodnan GP, Medsger TA Jr, Short D: Eosinophilic fasciitis: A pathologic study of twenty cases. *Am J Pathol* 96:493–518, 1979.

Belongia EA, Hedberg CW, Gleich GJ, et al: An investigation into the cause of the eosinophilia-myalgia syndrome. *N Engl J Med* 323:357–365, 1990.

Berger PB, Duffy J, Reeder GS, et al: Restrictive cardiomyopathy associated with the eosinophilia-myalgia syndrome. *Mayo Clin Proc* 69:162–165, 1994.

Campagna AC, Blanc PD, Criswell LA, et al: Pulmonary manifestations of the eosinophilic-myalgia syndrome associated with tryptophan ingestion. *Chest* 101: 1274–1281, 1992.

Doyle JA, Ginsburg WW: Eosinophilic fasciitis. *Med Clin North Am* 73:1157–1166, 1989.

Freundlich B, Werth VP, Rook AH, et al: L-tryptophan ingestion associated with eosinophilic fasciitis but not progressive systemic sclerosis. *Ann Intern Med* 112:758–762, 1990.

Gomez-Sanchez MA, Mestre de Juan MJ, Gomez-Pajuelo C, et al: Pulmonary hypertension due to toxic oil syndrome: A clinicopathologic study. *Chest* 95: 325–331, 1989

Gomez-Sanchez MA, Saenz de la Calzada C, Gomez-

Pajuelo C, et al: Clinical and pathologic manifestations of pulmonary vascular disease in toxic oil syndrome. *J Am Coll Cardiol* 18:1539–1545, 1991.

Grisanti MW, Moore TL, Osborn TG, Haber PL: Eosinophilic fasciitis in children. *Semin Arthritis Rheum* 19:151–157, 1989.

Herrick MK, Chang Y, Horoupian DS, et al: L-tryptophan and the eosinophilia-myalgia syndrome: Pathologic findings in eight patients. *Hum Pathol* 22: 12–21, 1991.

Hertzman PA, Borda IA: The toxic oil syndrome and the eosinophilia-myalgia syndrome: Pursuing clinical parallels. *J Rheumatol* 20:1707–1710, 1993.

Hertzman PA, Maddoux GL, Sternberg EM, et al: Repeated coronary artery spasm in a young woman with the eosinophilia-myalgia syndrome. *JAMA* 267: 2932–2934, 1992.

Hertzman PA, Falk H, Kilbourne EM, et al: The eosinophilia-myalgia syndrome: The Los Alamos Conference. *J Rheumatol* 18:867–873, 1991.

Hibbs JR, Mittleman B, Hill P, Medsger TA Jr: L-tryptophan-associated eosinophilic fasciitis prior to the 1989 eosinophilia-myalgia syndrome outbreak. *Arthritis Rheum* 35:299–303, 1992

James TN: The toxic oil syndrome. *Clin Cardiol* 17: 463–470, 1994.

James TN, Gomez-Sanchez A, Martinez-Tello, et al: Cardiac abnormalities in the toxic oil syndrome with comparative observations on the eosinophilia-myalgia syndrome. *J Am Coll Cardiol* 18:1367–1379, 1991.

James TN, Kamb ML, Sandberg GA, et al: Postmortem studies of the heart in three fatal cases of the eosinophilia-myalgia syndrome. *Ann Intern Med* 115:102–110, 1991.

James TN, Posada de la Paz M, Abaitua-Borda I, et al: Histologic abnormalities of large and small coronary arteries, neural structures, and the conduction system of the heart found in postmortem studies of individuals dying from the toxic oil syndrome. *Am Heart J* 121:803–815, 1991.

Kaufman LD: Eosinophilia-myalgia syndrome: Mortality and morbidity. *J Rheumatol* 20:1644–1646, 1993.

Kaufman LD: The evolving spectrum of eosinophilia-myalgia syndrome. *Rheum Dis Clin North Am* 20: 973–994, 1994.

Kaufman LD, Gruber BL, Gregerson PK: Clinical follow-up and immunogenetic studies of 32 patients with the eosinophilia-myalgia syndrome. *Lancet* 337: 1071–1074, 1991.

Kaufman LD, Kephart GM, Seidman RJ, et al: The spectrum of eosinophilic myositis: Clinical and immunopathogenic studies of three patients and review of the literature. *Arthritis Rheum* 36: 1014–1024, 1993.

Kaufman LD, Krupp LB: Eosinophilia-myalgia syndrome, toxic oil syndrome, and diffuse fasciitis with eosinophilia. *Curr Opin Rheumatol* 7:560–567, 1995.

Kent LT, Cramer SF, Moskowitz RW: Eosinophilic fasciitis: Clinical, laboratory, and microscopic considerations. *Arthritis Rheum* 24:677–683, 1981.

Kilbourne EM, de la Paz MP, Borda IB, et al: Toxic oil syndrome: A current clinical and epidemiologic summary, including comparison with the eosinophilia-myalgia syndrome. *J Am Coll Cardiol* 18:711–717, 1991.

Lakhanpal S, Ginsburg WW, Michet CJ, et al: Eosinophilic fasciitis: Clinical spectrum and therapeutic response in 52 cases. *Semin Arthritis Rheum* 17:221–231, 1988.

Levine B, Lanza DC, Ficco A, Freundlich B: Head and neck manifestations of eosinophilia-myalgia syndrome. *Ann Oto Rhino Laryngol* 104:90–99, 1995.

Lewkonia RM, Marx LH, Atkinson MH: Granulomatous vasculitis in the syndrome of diffuse fasciitis with eosinophilia. *Arch Intern Med* 142:73–75, 1982.

Lin JD, Phelps RG, Gordon ML, et al: Pathological manifestations of the eosinophilia myalgia syndrome: Analysis of 11 cases. *Hum Pathol* 23:429–437, 1992.

Lynn J, Rammohan KW, Bornstein RA, et al: Central nervous system involvement in the eosinophilia-myalgia syndrome. *Arch Neurol* 49:1082–1085, 1992.

Mar KE, Sen P, Tan K, et al: Bronchiolitis obliterans organizing pneumonia associated with massive L-Tryptophan ingestion. *Chest* 104:1924–1926, 1993.

Markusse HM, Dijmans BAC, Fibbe WE: Eosinophilic fasciitis after allogenic bone marrow transplantation. *J Rheumatol* 17:692–694, 1990.

Martin RW, Duffy J, Lie JT: Eosinophilic fasciitis associated with use of L-tryptophan: A case control study and comparison of clinical and histopathologic features. *Mayo Clin Proc* 66:892–898, 1991.

Martin RW, Duffy J, Lie JT, et al: The clinical spectrum of the eosinophilia-myalgia syndrome associated with L-tryptophan ingestion: Clinical features in 20 patients and aspects of pathophysiology. *Ann Intern Med* 113:124–134, 1990.

Martinez-Tello FJ, Navas-Palacios JJ, Ricoy JR, et al: Pathology of a new toxic oil syndrome caused by ingestion of adulterated oil in Spain. *Virchows Arch Pathol Anat* 397:261–285, 1982.

Oursler JR, Farmer ER, Roubenoff R, et al: Cutaneous manifestations of the eosinophilia-myalgia syndrome. *Br J Dermatol* 127:138–146, 1992.

Philen RM, Hill RH Jr, Flanders WD, et al: Tryptophan contaminants associated with eosinophilia-myalgia syndrome. *Am J Epidemiol* 138:154–159, 1993.

Philen RM, Posada M: Toxic oil syndrome and eosinophilia-myalgia syndrome: May 8–10, 1991, World Health Organization report. *Semin Arthritis Rheum* 23:104–124, 1993.

Rodnan GP, Dibartolomeo AG, Medsger TA Jr, et al: Eosinophilic fasciitis: Report of 7 cases of a newly recognized scleroderma-like syndrome. *Arthritis Rheum* 18:422–423, 1975.

Shulman LE: Diffuse fasciitis with hypergammaglobulinemia and eosinophilia: A new syndrome? *J Rheumatol* 1 (suppl 1):46, 1974.

Shulman LE: Diffuse fasciitis with eosinophilia: A new syndrome? *Trans Assoc Am Physicians* 88:70–85, 1975.

Shulman LE: The eosinophilia-myalgia syndrome associated with ingestion of L-Tryptophan. *Arthritis Rheum* 33:913–917, 1990.

Silver RM, Heyes MP, Maize JC, et al: Scleroderma, fasciitis, and eosinophilia associated with the ingestion of tryptophan. *N Engl J Med* 322:874–881, 1990.

Slutsker L, Hoesly FC, Miller L, et al: Eosinophilia-myalgia syndrome associated with exposure to tryptophan from a single manufacturer. *JAMA* 264:213–217, 1990.

Smith BE, Dyck PJ: Peripheral neuropathy in the eosinophilia-myalgia syndrome associated with L-tryptophan ingestion. *Neurology* 40:1035–1040, 1990.

Spinner RJ, Ginsburg WW, Lie JT, et al: Atypical eosinophilic fasciitis localized to the hands and feet: A report of four cases. *J Rheumatol* 19:1141–1146, 1992.

Spitzer WO, Haggerty JL, Berkson L, et al: Continuing occurrence of eosinophilia-myalgia syndrome in Canada. *Br J Rheumatol* 34:246–251, 1995.

Swygert LA, Back EE, Auerbach SB, et al: Eosinophilia-myalgia syndrome: Mortality data from the U.S. national surveillance system. *J Rheumatol* 20: 1711–1717, 1993.

Swygert LA, Maes EF, Sewell LE, et al: Eosinophilia-myalgia syndrome: Results of national surveillance. *JAMA* 264:1698–1703, 1990.

Tazelaar HD, Myers JL, Drage CW, et al: Pulmonary disease associated with L-tryptophan-induced eosinophilia-myalgia syndrome. *Chest* 97:1032–1036, 1990.

Tazelaar HD, Myers JL, Strikler JG, et al: Tryptophan-induced lung disease: An immuno-phenotypic, immunofluorescent, and electron microscopic study. *Mod Pathol* 6:56–60, 1993.

Thacker HL: Eosinophilia-myalgia syndrome: The Cleveland Clinic experience. *Cleve Clin J Med* 58: 400–408, 1991.

Toxic Epidemic Syndrome Study Group: Toxic epidemic syndrome, Spain, 1981. *Lancet* 2:697–702, 1982.

Travis WD, Kalafer ME, Robin HS, et al: Hypersensitivity pneumonitis and pulmonary vasculitis with eosinophilia in a patient taking an L-tryptophan preparation. *Ann Intern Med* 112:301–303, 1990.

Van den Bergh V, Tricot G, Fonteyn G, et al: Diffuse fasciitis after bone marrow transplantation. *Am J Med* 83:39–143, 1987.

Varga J, Heiman-Patterson TD, Emergy DL, et al: Clinical spectrum of the systemic manifestations of the eosinophilia-myalgia syndrome. *Semin Arthritis Rheum* 19:313–328, 1990.

Verity MA, Bulpitt KJ, Paulus HE: Neuromuscular manifestations of L-tryptophan-associated eosinophilia-myalgia syndrome: A histomorphologic analysis of 14 patients. *Hum Pathol* 22:3–11, 1991.

Williamson MR, Eidson M, Rosenberg RD, et al: Eosinophilia-myalgia syndrome: Findings on chest radiographs in 18 patients. *Radiology* 180:849–852, 1991.

Winkelmann RK, Connolly SM, Quimby SR, Lie JT, et al: Histopathologic features of the L-tryptophan related eosinophilia myalgia (fasciitis) syndrome. *Mayo Clin Proc* 66:457–463, 1991.

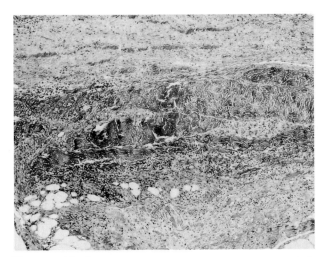

Figure 15.1. Thickened deep fascia in eosinophilic fasciitis with edema and a lymphoplasmacytic infiltrate containing many eosinophils.

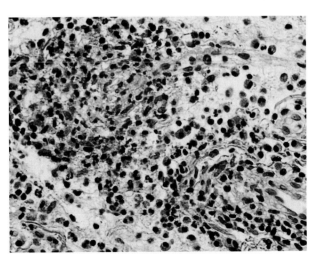

Figure 15.2. Close-up view at higher magnification of eosinophils in the inflammatory infiltrate of eosinophilic fasciitis.

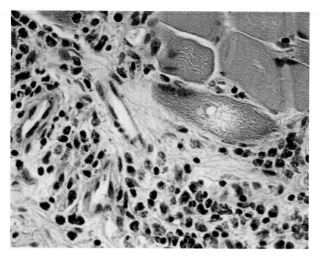

Figure 15.3. Eosinophilic myositis with perimysial inflammatory infiltrate in EMS.

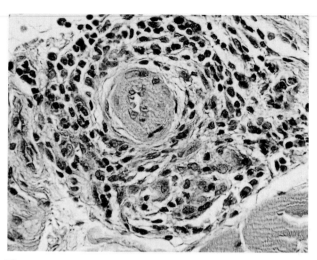

Figure 15.4. Small-vessel eosinophilic perivascular infiltrate in a muscle biopsy of EMS.

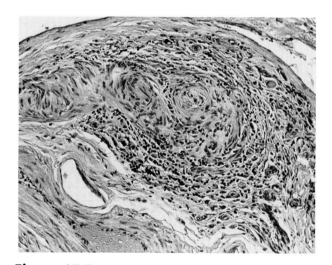

Figure 15.5. Small-vessel vasculitis in a sural nerve biopsy of EMS.

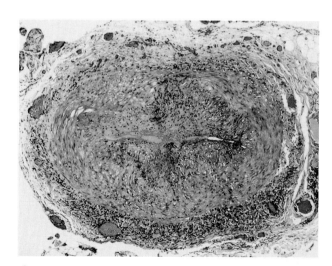

Figure 15.6. Non-giant cell eosinophilic temporal arteritis in a 57-year-old woman with EMS.

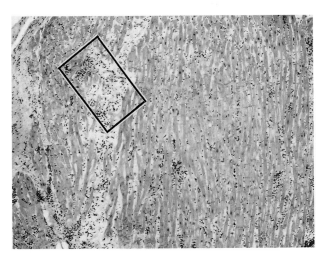

Figure 15.7. Diagnosis of myocarditis by endomyocardial biopsy in a 38-year-old woman with EMS and otherwise unexplained heart failure.

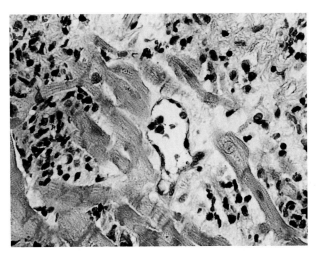

Figure 15.8. Close-up view at higher magnification of eosinophilic myocarditis in the boxed area of **Fig. 15.7.**

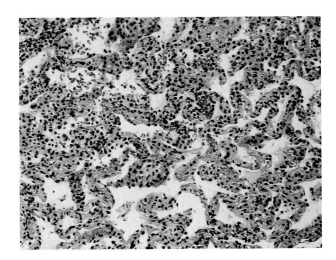

Figure 15.9. Open-lung biopsy showing hypersensitivity pneumonitis with eosinophilic infiltrate in EMS.

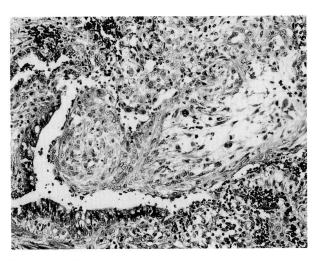

Figure 15.10. Open-lung biopsy showing bronchiolitis obliterans in a patient with EMS.

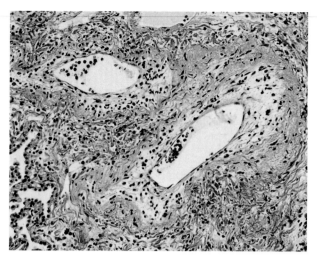

Figure 15.11. Open-lung biopsy showing eosinophilic pulmonary vasculitis in a patient with EMS.

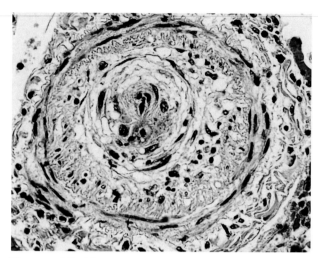

Figure 15.12. Open-lung biopsy showing proliferative vaso-occlusive disease of pulmonary hypertension in a patient with EMS.

16. Familial Mediterranean Fever

Also known as "recurrent hereditary polyserositis," familial Mediterranean fever (FMF) is an autosomal recessively inherited disorder characterized by recurrent attacks of inflammation involving, principally, the peritoneum, pleura, synovia, and skin. Peritoneal and synovial fluids of patients with FMF lack a protein that inhibits neutrophil chemotaxis by antagonizing the complement-derived inflammatory mediator C5a. The absent C5a inhibitor activity may be related to a genetic defect in one of the family of lipocortin proteins, because there is evidence supporting an abnormality in the first step of prostaglandin/leukotriene synthesis in FMF patients.

It seems possible that autoimmune features observed in FMF are nonspecific changes of inflammation and not due to autoimmune mechanisms. A recent serologic survey of several hundreds of Israeli FMF patients and their first degree relatives found no evidence of increased incidence of autoantibodies to ssDNA, dsDNA, poly (I), poly (G), cardiolipin, histones, RNP and Ro(SSA), when compared to healthy controls.

FMF occurs predominantly in persons living in or originating from the Mediterranean shores, especially people of Jewish (Sephardic more commonly than Ashkenazic ancestry), Arabian, Turkish, and Armenian descent. The disease is seldom encountered outside the Mediterranean countries except among the emigrants or travelers from that region.

FMF is essentially a disease of children and young adults. Because of its protean clinical manifestations, the diagnosis of the disease outside the Mediterranean countries requires a high degree of clinical acuity, especially when key laboratory test abnormalities may be limited to elevated erythrocyte sedimentation rate and joint fluid leukocyte counts during attacks. The major cause of death among adult patients with FMF is amyloidosis and its complications, especially renal amyloidosis. Colchicine is usually effective in preventing progressive renal damage in FMF.

Biopsy diagnosis of FMF centers around the detection of amyloidosis. A major problem in making an antemortem diagnosis of FMF relates to the peculiar tissue distribution of the amyloid deposits. Analysis of the fat aspirate and bone marrow and/or lymphnode biopsy specimens is unlikely to reveal amyloid deposits in FMF, in contrast to other types of primary amyloidosis (AL amyloid), reactive amyloidosis (AA amyloid), or hereditary amyloidosis (AF amyloid). A rectal or liver biopsy (Fig. 16.1) is more likely to be positive for amyloidosis in the early stage of FMF but when the disease is well established and the patient is in renal failure, the renal biopsy is almost invariably positive for amyloid deposits (Fig. 16.2). A rare renal manifestation of FMF is crescentic rapidly progressive glomerulonephritis without amyloidosis (Fig. 16.3), which was first reported by Said et al in 1989.

Cardiac or pulmonary amyloidosis also occurs in patients with FMF, and may be detectable in an endomyocardial (Fig. 16.4) or open lung (Fig. 16.5) biopsy, respectively. In both of these locations, the amyloid deposits are predominantly vascular rather than interstitial in distribution. Unexplained heart failure, cardiac arrhythmia, or pulmonary disease in patients known to have FMF is an indication for a diagnostic endomyocardial or open lung biopsy. Of considerable interest, a previously unknown or unrecognized pulmonary hypertension due to amyloidosis of the lung in FMF (Fig. 16.6) was first described by Johnson and Lie in 1991.

A polyarteritis nodosa (PAN) type necrotizing vasculitis occurs in FMF patients significantly more often than the reported general population incidence of about 6 per 100,000. Among the 20 or so reported cases, the mean age of onset of PAN in FMF was 21 years, which is considerably younger than that of PAN in the general population (45 years). Most clinical manifestations of PAN in FMF patients resemble those of PAN in general, except that subcutaneous nodules and myalgia occur twice as commonly as they do in the classic PAN. Diagnosis is by muscle biopsy.

BIBLIOGRAPHY

Ben-Chetrit E, Levy M: Colchicine prophylaxis in familial Mediterranean fever: Reappraisal after 15 years. *Semin Arthritis Rheum* 20:241–246, 1991.

Eliakim M, Rachmilewitz M, Rosenmann E, Niv A: Renal manifestations in recurrent polyserositis (familial Mediterranean fever). *Isr J Med Sci* 6:228–245, 1970.

Gafni J, Ravid M, Sohar E: The role of amyloidosis in familial Mediterranean fever: A population study. *Isr J Med Sci* 4:995–999, 1968.

Glikson M, Galun E, Schlesinger M, et al: Polyarteritis nodosa and familial Mediterranean fever: A report of 2 cases and review of the literature. *J Rheumatol* 16: 536–539, 1989.

Goldfinger SE: Familial Mediterranean fever—An

update. *Trans Am Clin Climatol Assoc* 98:128–132, 1986.

Johnson WJ, Lie JT: Pulmonary hypertension and familial Mediterranean fever: A previously unrecognized association. *Mayo Clin Proc* 66:919–925, 1991.

Majeed HA, Barakat M: Familial Mediterranean fever (recurrent hereditary polyserositis) in children: Analysis of 88 cases. *Eur J Pediatr* 148:636–641, 1989.

Matzner Y: Familial Mediterranean fever—An autoimmune disorder or a genetic defect in a regulatory mechanism of inflammation. *Isr J Med Sci* 25:547–549, 1989.

Matzner Y, Ayesh SK, Hochner-Celniker D, et al: Proposed mechanism of the inflammatory attacks in familial Mediterranean fever. *Arch Intern Med* 150:1289–1291, 1990.

Moore PJ, Mansour A, McDonald JD, et al: Familial Mediterranean fever in six Australian children. *Med J Aust* 151:108–110, 1989.

Mornaghi R, Rubinstein P, Franklin EC: Familial Mediterranean amyloidosis: Case reports and genetic studies. *Am J Med* 73:609–614, 1982.

Pras M, Langevitz P, Livneh A, Zemer D: Vasculitis in familial Mediterranean fever. In Ansell BM, Bacon PA, Lie JT, Yazici H (eds): *The Vasculitides: Science and Practice.* London, Chapman & Hall, 1996:412–416.

Rimon D, Meir Y, Cohen L: Retroperitoneal lymphadenopathy in familial Mediterranean fever. *Postgrad Med J* 65:776–778, 1989.

Said R, Hamzeh Y, Tarawneh M, et al: Rapid progressive glomerulonephritis in patients with familial Mediterranean fever. *Am J Kid Dis* 14:412–416, 1989.

Shiue ST, McNally DP: Pulmonary hypertension from prominent vascular involvement in diffuse amyloidosis. *Arch Intern Med* 148:687–689, 1988.

Shohat M, Korenberg JR, Schwabe AD, Rotter JI: Hypothesis: Familial Mediterranean fever—A genetic disorder of the lipocortin family? *Am J Med Genet* 34:163–167, 1989.

Sohar E, Gafni J, Pras M, Heller H: Familial Mediterranean fever: A survey of 470 cases and review of the literature. *Am J Med* 43:227–253, 1967.

Swissa M, Schul V, Korish S, et al: Determination of autoantibodies in patients with familial Mediterranean fever and their first degree relatives. *J Rheumatol* 18:606–608, 1991.

Tishler M, Pras M, Yaron M: Abdominal fat tissue aspirate in amyloidosis of familial Mediterranean fever. *Clin Exp Rheumatol* 6:395–397, 1988.

Zemer D, Livneh A, Danon YL, et al: Long-term colchicine treatment in children with familial Mediterranean fever. *Arthritis Rheum* 34:973–977, 1991.

Zemer D, Pras M, Sohar E, et al: Colchicine in prevention and treatment of amyloidosis of familial Mediterranean fever. *N Engl J Med* 314:1001–1005, 1986.

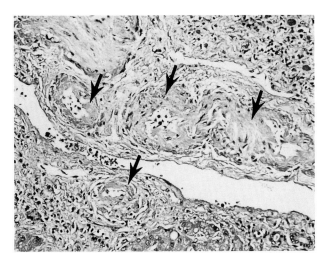

Figure 16.1. Vascular amyloidosis (*arrows*) in the liver biopsy of a young patient with FMF.

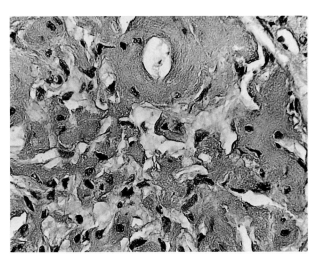

Figure 16.2. Diffuse and heavy glomerular amyloid deposits in renal biopsy of a FMF patient.

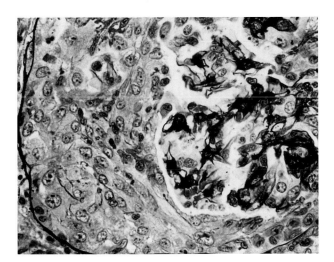

Figure 16.3. Crescentic rapidly progressive glomerulonephritis in renal biopsy of a FMF patient.

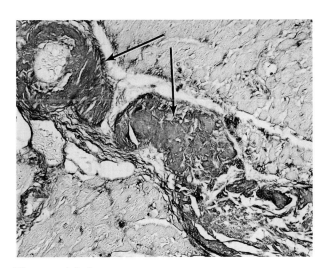

Figure 16.4. Vascular amyloid deposits (*arrows*) in endomyocardial biopsy of a FMF patient.

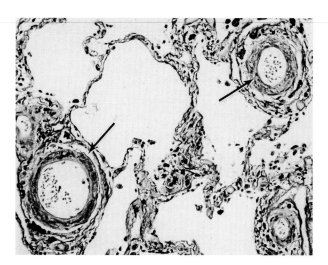

Figure 16.5. Vascular amyloid deposits (*arrows*) in open lung biopsy of a FMF patient.

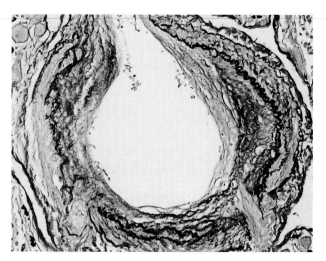

Figure 16.6. Proliferative vaso-occlusive disease in a FMF patient with pulmonary hypertension.

17. Kawasaki Disease

WHAT IS KAWASAKI DISEASE?

Also known as Kawasaki syndrome, Kawasaki disease is an infantile febrile illness of unknown cause; the disease is recognized by the presence of any five of the six principal clinical manifestations based on the 1984 revised diagnostic guidelines prepared and published by the *Japan Kawasaki Disease Research Committee:*

1. Fever persisting for 5 days or longer.
2. Reddening of palms and soles, with brawny indurative edema in initial stage and membranous desquamation of the finger tips in the convalescent phase.
3. Polymorphous exanthema.
4. Bilateral conjunctivitis.
5. Reddening of lips and oropharyngeal mucosa, strawberry tongue.
6. Acute non-suppurative cervical lymphadenopathy.

Patients with only four of the above six items can be diagnosed in the presence of coronary artery aneurysms or arteritis, which occur in 15 to 30% of cases. Some investigators consider the above diagnostic guidelines too strict and suggest that cases not fulfilling the above criteria (so-called atypical Kawasaki disease) be treated the same as typical Kawasaki disease because of the same high and potentially life-threatening complication rate.

Kawasaki disease is not new or rare. It was initially described as the "mucocutaneous lymph node syndrome" in 1967 in Japan and later in the English-language literature in 1974 by the Japanese pediatrician Tomisaku Kawasaki. Within the next 10 years, well over 80,000 cases had been reported in Japan alone. However, as early as in the late 1930s through mid-1960s, sporadic cases clinically strikingly similar to patients who die of Kawasaki disease were reported in the English-language literature as *infantile polyarteritis nodosa* with multiple vascular lesions histologically indistinguishable from those seen in the 2% fatal cases of Kawasaki disease.

Kawasaki disease has a worldwide distribution, affecting predominantly infants and young children under five years of age with a male preponderance. There is an ethnic bias towards Oriental or Afro-Caribbean children, some seasonality and occasional epidemics. In Japanese populations, the incidence is 150 per 100,000 per year for children aged five years or younger. Elsewhere, the incidence is significantly lower: 10.3 per 100,000 per year in the United States, and about 3 per 100,000 per year in several European countries including the United Kingdom, for children under five years of age. The familial second-case rate for siblings is 2.1% in Japan.

After Schönlein-Henoch syndrome, Kawasaki disease ranks as the next most common form of childhood vasculitis. Rarely, Kawasaki disease may coexist with systemic lupus erythematosus. Sudden unexpected death may occur in infancy at the acute phase of the disease from ruptured coronary artery aneurysms or fulminant myocarditis, or in adolescents and young adults as late sequelae of coronary arteritis or occluded coronary aneurysms by thrombosis or fibrous intimal proliferation, with or without myocardial infarction. Recurrences of the disease may also occur.

Kawasaki disease is said to be unsafe at any age because of the serious and potentially life-threatening late sequelae. The possibility of atherosclerotic lesions in adults secondary to previous damage of the coronary arteries from childhood Kawasaki disease also needs to be considered. Coronary arteritis can cause endothelial damage and may lead to lipid insudation into the vascular wall. Although there is no clear evidence to predict premature atherosclerotic coronary artery disease in Kawasaki disease patients with resolved aneurysms, the known mechanism of aneurysm healing and repair process by fibrosis would suggest some increased risk, especially among those individuals who have other independent risk factors for atherosclerosis.

HOW MAY THE DIAGNOSIS OF KAWASAKI DISEASE BE VERIFIED?

Whether the high frequency of Kawasaki disease in Japan is due to genetic or environmental influence is unknown. Several unconfirmed studies have associated Kawasaki disease with histocompatibility antigens: HLA-Bw22 in Japanese and Bw51 or combined A2, B44, Cw5 in North American patients.

Results of laboratory tests in Kawasaki disease are nonspecific but useful. Investigations may reveal a polymorphonuclear leukocytosis, thrombocythemia, elevated acute-phase protein and erythrocyte sedimentation rate, circulating immune complexes and both antineutrophil cytoplasmic antibodies (ANCA) and antiendothelial cell antibodies. The ANCA on immunofluorescence are said to be very characteristic, with a *diffuse* cytoplasmic staining that is distinct from the *granular* cytoplasmic staining pattern seen in Wegener's granulomatosis or the *perinuclear* pattern in renal-associated disease and other non-Wegener's vasculitides. Coronary arterial aneurysms, when present, may be diagnosed by two-dimensional echocardiography or coronary angiography.

Careful analysis of autopsy materials by Japanese investigators (Fujiwara et al. 1988) have documented four stages in the pathology of coronary artery lesions in Kawasaki disease. Acute inflammatory changes are seen in the first 6 to 9 days in the intima and adventitia, progressing to the media to become transmural by 12 to 25 days. Aneurysms appear subsequently by 28 to 32 days, but may be as early as within the first two weeks of the early phase of the disease. Marked stenosis following recanalization of organized thrombi and post-repair intimal fibrosis are seen after 40 days. The previously dilated aneurysmal lumen becomes gradually filled-in by intimal fibrosis, producing what appears angiographically to be a resolution or regression of the aneurysm when in reality a transformation of the dilated coronary artery to a stiffer, noncompliant, and progressively more obstructive coronary artery.

Biopsy diagnosis of Kawasaki disease is limited to special selected circumstances. The all important and potentially lethal epicardial large-vessel coronary arteritis and aneurysms are virtually never biopsied except at surgical intervention for complications, such as rupture. The angiographic evidence for regression or resolution of coronary aneurysms is based on restoration to near-normal caliber of the previously dilated arterial lumen following post-repair fibrocellular intimal proliferation (FIP). The post-repair FIP may, on the other hand, cause vaso-occlusive disease of the coronary artery that necessitates bypass or interposition grafting and thereby makes available an excised segment of the obstructed coronary artery for biopsy diagnosis (Fig. 17.1).

Japanese investigators also have extensive experience of endomyocardial biopsies in patients with Kawasaki disease. In a large series of 201 children, age one month to 11 years, all of whom underwent diagnostic coronary angiography and endomyocardial biopsy, Yutani et al. (1981) found aneurysms of major branches of the coronary arteries in 26 (13%) of the 201 children, and they also found "myocarditis, cellular infiltration, and fibrosis in every case." In our more restricted experience with pediatric patients in North America, we have also observed both necrotizing myocarditis (Fig. 17.2) and intramural coronary vasculitis (Fig. 17. 3) in 6 of 9 chil-

dren under 12 years of age who underwent diagnostic endomyocardial biopsy for an otherwise unexplained acute-onset heart failure at early stage of Kawasaki disease.

Other more infrequent biopsy confirmation of extracardiac manifestations of Kawasaki disease include polyarteritis-type vasculitis in renal biopsy (Fig. 17.4), liver biopsy (Fig. 17.5), and sural nerve biopsy (Fig. 17.6). Only angiographic evidence of cerebral involvement has been reported. In our experience, skeletal muscle biopsies have not been very helpful; they tend to show nonspecific interstitial or perivascular inflammatory cell infiltrate rather than a true vasculitis. There is an unconfirmed report of the utility of lymph node biopsy in Kawasaki disease (Giesker et al. 1982).

BIBLIOGRAPHY

Aballi AJ: Kawasaki disease. *Int Pediatr* 1:44–52, 1986.

Albat B, Missov E, Leclercq F, et al: Adult coronary aneurysm related to Kawasaki disease. *J Cardiovasc Surg* 35:57–60, 1994.

Burns JC, Shike H, Gordon JB, et al: Sequelae of Kawasaki disease in adolescents and young adults. *J Am Coll Cardiol* 28:253–257, 1996.

Butler DF, Hough DR, Friedman SJ, Davis HE: Adult Kawasaki disease. Arch *Dermatol* 123:1356–1361, 1987.

Dillon MJ: Kawasaki syndrome. In Ansell BM, Bacon PA, Lie JT, Yazici H (eds): *The Vasculitides: Science and Practice.* London, Chapman & Hall, 1996: 384–391.

Ettlinger RE, Nelson AM, Burke EC, Lie JT: Polyarteritis nodosa in childhood: A clinical pathologic study. *Arthritis Rheum* 22:820–825, 1979.

Flugelman MY, Hasin Y, Basfan MM, et al: Acute myocardial infarction 14 years after an acute episode of Kawasaki's disease. *Am J Cardiol* 52:427–433, 1983.

Fujiwara T, Fujiwara H, Kakano H: Pathological features of coronary arteries in children with Kawasaki disease in which coronary arterial aneurysm was absent at autopsy. *Circulation* 78:345–350, 1988.

Fujita Y, Nakamura Y, Sakata K, et al: Kawasaki disease in families. *Pediatrics* 84:666–669, 1989.

Gersony WM: Diagnosis and management of Kawasaki disease. *JAMA* 265:2699–2703, 1991.

Giesker DW, Pastuszak WT, Forouhar FA, et al: Lymph node biopsy for early diagnosis in Kawasaki disease. *Am J Surg Pathol* 6:493–501, 1982.

Japan Kawasaki Disease Research Committee: *Diagnostic Guidelines of Kawasaki Disease,* ed 4. Tokyo, Japan Red Cross Medical Center, 1984.

Joffe A, Kabani A, Jadavji T: Atypical and complicated Kawasaki disease in infants: Do we need criteria? *West J Med* 162:322–327, 1995.

Kaslow RA, Bailowitz A, Lin FYC, et al: Association of epidemic Kawasaki syndrome with the HLA-A2, B44, Cw5 antigen combination. *Arthritis Rheum* 28: 938–940, 1985.

Kato S, Kimura M, Tsuji K, et al: HLA antigen in Kawasaki disease. *Pediatrics* 61:252–255, 1978.

Kawasaki T: Mucocutaneous lymph node syndrome: Clinical observation of 50 cases. *Jap J Allergy* 16: 178–222, 1967 [in Japanese].

Kawasaki T, Kosaki F, Okawa S, et al: A new infantile febrile mucocutaneous lymph node syndrome (MLNS) prevailing in Japan. *Pediatrics* 54:271–276, 1974.

Landing BH, Larson EJ: Pathological features of Kawasaki disease (mucocutaneous lymph node syndrome). *Am J Surg Pathol* 1:215–229, 1987.

Lapointe JS, Nugent RA, Graeb DA, Robertson WD: Cerebral infarction and regression of widespread aneurysms in Kawasaki's disease: Case report. *Pediatr Radiol* 14:1–5, 1984.

Laxer RM, Cameron BJ, Silverman ED: Occurrence of Kawasaki disease and systemic lupus erythematosus in a single patient. *J Rheumatol* 15:515–516, 1988.

Leung DYM: Immunologic aspects of Kawasaki disease. *J Rheumatol* 17 (suppl 24):15–18, 1990.

Lie JT: Infantile polyarteritis and fatal cases of Kawasaki syndrome: Two diseases or one? In Shulman ST (ed): *Kawasaki Disease: Proceedings of the Second International Kawasaki Disease Symposium.* New York, Alan R. Liss, 1987:521.

Meissner HC, Leung DYM: Kawasaki syndrome. *Curr Opin Rheumatol* 7:455–458, 1995.

Melish ME, Hicks RV: Kawasaki syndrome: Clinical features, pathophysiology, etiology and therapy. *J Rheumatol* 17 (suppl 24):2–10, 1990.

Michels TC: Mucocutaneous lymph node syndrome in adults: Differentiation from toxic shock syndrome. *Am J Med* 80:724–728, 1986.

Nakamura Y, Yanagawa H, Kawasaki T: Mortality among children with Kawasaki disease in Japan. *N Engl J Med* 326:1246–1249, 1992.

Naoe S, Takahashi, Masuda H, Tanaka N: Kawasaki disease: With particular emphasis on arterial lesions. *Acta Pathol Jpn* 41:785–797, 1991.

Onouchi Z, Hamaoka K, Kamiya Y, et al: Transformation of coronary artery aneurysm to obstructive lesion in patients with Kawasaki disease. *J Am Coll Cardiol* 21:158–162, 1993.

Rose V: Kawasaki syndrome: Cardiovascular manifestations. *J Rheumatol* 17 (suppl 24):11–14, 1990.

Ross BA: Kawasaki disease: Unsafe at any age. *J Am Coll Cardiol* 25 1425–1427, 1995.

Sasaguri Y, Kato H: Regression of aneurysms in Kawasaki disease: A pathological study. *J Pediatr* 100:225–231, 1982.

Savage COS, Tizard EJ, Jayne D, et al: Antineutrophil cytoplasmic antibodies in Kawasaki disease. *Arch Dis Child* 64:360–363, 1989.

Suzuki A, Kamiya T, Kuwahara N, et al: Coronary arterial lesions of Kawasaki disease: Cardiac catheterization findings of 1100 cases. *Pediatr Cardiol* 7:3–9, 1986.

Suzuki A, Kamiya T, Ono Y, et al: Myocardial ischemia in Kawasaki disease: Follow-up study by cardiac catheterization and coronary angiography. *Pediatr Cardiol* 9:1–5, 1988.

Takahashi M: Myocarditis in Kawasaki syndrome: A minor villain? *Circulation* 79:1398–1400, 1989.

Tanaka N, Naoe S, Masuda H, Ueno T: Pathological study of sequelae of Kawasaki disease (MCLS): With special reference to the heart and coronary arterial lesions. *Acta Pathol Jpn* 36:1513–1547, 1986.

Tanaka N, Sekimoto K, Naoe S: Kawasaki disease: Relationship with infantile polyarteritis nodosa. *Arch Pathol Lab Med* 100:81–86, 1976.

Tatara K, Kusakawa S, Itoh K, et al: Long-term prognosis of Kawasaki disease patients with coronary artery obstruction. *Heart Vessels* 5:47–51, 1989.

Tizard EJ, Baguley E, Hughes GRV, Dillon MJ: Antiendothelial cell antibodies detected by a cellular based ELIZA in Kawasaki disease. *Arch Dis Child* 66: 189–192, 1991.

Tizard EJ, Suzuki A, Levin M, Dillon MJ: Clinical aspects of 100 patients with Kawasaki disease. *Arch Dis Child* 66:185–188, 1991.

Vargo TA, Huhta JC, Moore WH, Person DA: Recurrent Kawasaki disease. *Pediatr Cardiol* 6:199–202, 1986.

Wortmann DW: Kawasaki disease. *Semin Arthritis Rheum* 11:37–47, 1992.

Wreford FS, Conradi SE, Cohle SD, Lie JT: Sudden death caused by coronary artery aneurysms: A late complication of Kawasaki disease. *J Forens Sci* 36:51–59, 1991.

Yanagawa H, Nakamura Y: Nationwide epidemic of Kawasaki disease in Japan during winter of 1985–1986. *Lancet* 2:1138–1140, 1986.

Yutani C, Go S, Kamiya T, et al: Cardiac biopsy of Kawasaki disease. *Arch Pathol Lab Med* 105:470–473, 1981.

Yutani C, Okano K, Kamiya T, et al: Histopathological study on right ventricular endomyocardial biopsy of Kawasaki disease. *Br Heart J* 43:589–592, 1980.

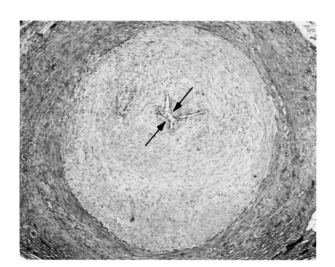

Figure 17.1. Late sequela of "healed" coronary artery aneurysm with marked fibrous intimal proliferation resulting in near-occlusion of the lumen (*arrows*).

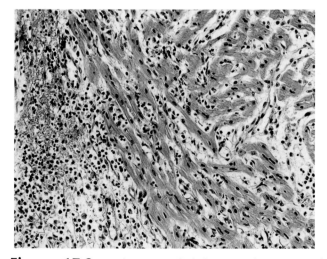

Figure 17.2. Endomyocardial biopsy diagnosis of necrotizing myocarditis in a 3-year-old boy with acute-phase Kawasaki disease.

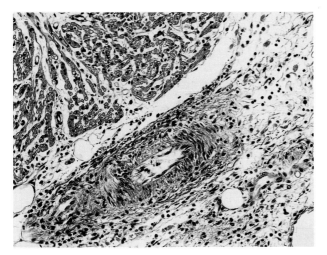

Figure 17.3. Vasculitis of a small intramural coronary artery in the same patient whose biopsy is shown in **Fig. 17.2.**

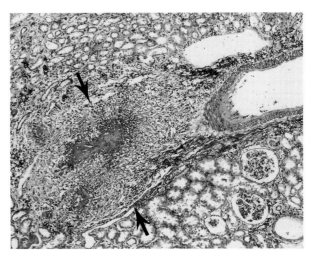

Figure 17.4. Polyarteritis-type necrotizing vasculitis of interlobar artery (*arrows*) in renal biopsy of a 6-year-old boy with Kawasaki disease.

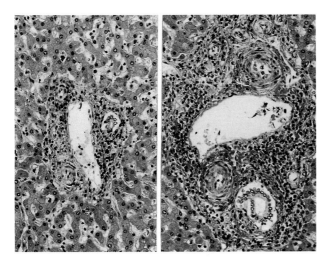

Figure 17.5. Liver biopsy in the same patient illustrated in **Fig. 17.4.** showing minimal (*left*) and unequivocal (*right*) evidence of arteriolar vasculitis in the portal tracts.

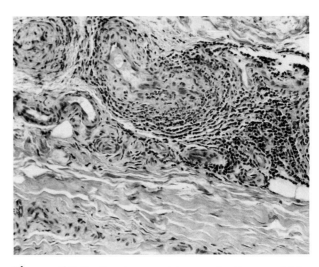

Figure 17.6. Sural nerve biopsy of a 9-year-old boy with Kawasaki disease showing a small vessel polyarteritis-type vasculitis.

18. Lyme Disease

CLINICAL DIAGNOSIS OF LYME DISEASE

Lyme disease, or Lyme borreliosis, is the most commonly recognized vector-born disease in the United States, having been reported in 43 states; its occurrence on five continents of the world also has been documented. The disease is caused by the *Treponema*-like spirochete *Borrelia burgdorferi* (*B burgdorferi*), which is transmitted to humans by the tick *Ixodes dammini*. Sporadic cases were first described in the northeastern United States as a new clinical entity in 1977 because of a clustering of affected children in the small community of Lyme, Connecticut, who were thought initially to have juvenile rheumatoid arthritis. In the two decades following its first description, Lyme disease has become endemic in many different geographic regions of the United States. Since 1982, some 20,000 cases of Lyme disease have been reported to the Centers for Disease Control; the annual incidence has increased almost tenfold from 492 cases in 1982 to 4,572 cases in 1988.

Lyme borreliosis is a systemic disease that may have dermatologic, rheumatologic, cardiac and neurologic manifestations at various clinical stages, but the pathognomonic feature of early Lyme disease is a distinctive skin rash or eruption known as *erythema chronicum migrans* (ECM), more recently as *erythema migrans* (EM). The three clinical stages covering the broad spectrum of Lyme disease roughly parallel their chronologic appearance, but overlap of stages is common and not all patients manifest signs and symptoms of each stage of the disease (Table 17.1).

The diagnosis of Lyme disease is based on clinical findings in most patients, especially those presenting with erythema migrans and/or a history of exposure to geographic locations endemic for the disease. Detection of a specific antibody to *B burgdorferi* is a useful confirmatory test in many patients. In clinically atypical cases of Lyme disease, a positive serologic test can be pivotal for the diagnosis and decision-making in instituting definitive treatment. However, serologic test results should not be used indiscriminately to diagnose Lyme disease, or as the sole basis for starting antibiotic therapy.

The presence of chronic Lyme disease cannot be excluded by the absence of antibodies against *B burgdorferi;* a specific T-cell blastogenic response to *B burgdorferi* is evidence of infection in the seronegative patients with clinical indications of chronic Lyme disease. A sensitive and direct diagnostic method capable of detecting *B burgdorferi* or *B burgdorferi*-specific components would improve the specificity for the diagnosis of Lyme disease. To this end, detection of *B burgdorferi* DNA by a polymerase chain reaction (PCR) method has proved useful. A strong correlation between the results of PCR and culture of tissues from experimentally infected mice has been documented recently. The results of another recent study suggest that detection of chromosomal *B burgdorferi* DNA may be more efficient in the synovial tissue than in the synovial fluid.

BIOPSY DIAGNOSIS OF LYME DISEASE

The role of biopsy diagnosis in Lyme disease has evolved languidly over the two decades after the initial description of the clinical entity because patients are not readily biopsied as a routine. The signs and symptoms of Lyme disease are generally transitory except for chronic and persistent involvement of the central and peripheral nervous system, joints and synovia. Involved sites in the body manifested by pain and swelling that are not routinely biopsied may include lymph nodes, liver, and gonads. Myocarditis in Lyme disease becomes increasingly recognized only by clinicians who actively seek it.

Table 18.1 Clinical Manifestations in Various Stages of Lyme Disease*

Stage	Clinical Manifestations
I	*Lasting a median of 4 weeks* ■ Erythema migrans ■ Influenza-like illness and fatigue ■ Musculoskeletal pains ■ Headache and stiffneck
II	*Lasting days to months* ■ Central nervous system disease: meningitis, encephalitis, Bell's palsy ■ Peripheral nervous system disease: radiculopathy or neuropathy or both ■ Cardiac involvement: arrhythmia, heart blocks, congestive heart failure ■ Ophthalmitis
III	*Lasting months to years* ■ Asymmetric pauciarticular arthritis, often intermittent but chronic in 10% of cases ■ Chronic, severe, late central nervous system disease: encephalitis, demyelinating syndromes, and psychiatric disorders

*Modified from Duffy J, et al. *Mayo Clin Proc* 1988;63:1116–1121.

181

For the great majority of patients, the diagnosis of Lyme disease is initiated by a high index of clinical suspicion, based on the history of exposure to or possible contact with the tick vectors and the characteristic skin rash, and subsequently supported by serologic testing or by PCR detection of *B burgdorferi* DNA in the body fluid or tissue.

Nevertheless, judiciously selected biopsies play an essential role in providing evidence for confirming the suspected systemic involvements in Lyme disease, many of which are chronically disabling to the patients, and some may be life threatening.

Up to 10% of untreated patients develop Lyme carditis at an average of 2 to 6 weeks after disease onset. With aggressive antibiotic therapy for early Lyme disease, carditis is observed most often in patients who had minimal or no symptoms associated with the onset of their infection and did not seek medical attention. Cardiac involvement in Lyme disease may be clinically silent and fatal. The common clinical presentations of Lyme carditis may include palpitations, arrhythmia, unexplained syncope, and various degrees of atrioventricular heart block. Lyme carditis is typically a nonspecific lymphoplasmacytic carditis and an endomyocardial biopsy is necessary for a definitive diagnosis (Fig. 18.1). Proof of *B burgdorferi* can be established by a positive culture of or the histological demonstration of the spirochetes.

Other biopsy-documented systemic involvements in Lyme disease include an inflammatory myopathy or myositis (Fig. 18.2), a rheumatoid arthritis-like synovitis (Fig. 18.3), and the rare case of necrotizing vasculitis found unexpectedly in a lymph node biopsy (Fig. 18.4). About 15% of untreated patients and patients who failed antibiotic therapy for early Lyme disease develop a wide spectrum of neurologic abnormalities that include meningitis, meningoencephalitis, cranial nerve palsies, radiculoneuritis, and peripheral neuritis. Brain biopsies in Lyme disease, to our knowledge, have not been undertaken. Peripheral nerve biopsies in symptomatic patients with Lyme disease may show a lymphocytic ganglioneuritis (Fig. 18.5) or a polyarteritis-type small vessel vasculitis (Fig. 18.6).

BIBLIOGRAPHY

Atlas E, Novak SN, Duray PH, Steere AC: Lyme myositis: Muscle invasion by *Borrelia burgdorferi*. *Ann Intern Med* 109:245–246, 1988.

Dattwyler RJ, Volkman DJ, Luft BJ, et al: Seronegative Lyme disease: Dissociation of specific T- and B-lymphocyte response to *Borrelia burgdorferi*. *N Engl J Med* 319:1441–1446, 1988.

Duffy J, Mertz LE, Wobig G, Katzmann JA: Diagnosing Lyme disease: The contribution of serologic testing. *Mayo Clin Proc* 63:1116–1121, 1988.

Duray PH: The surgical pathology of human Lyme disease: An enlarging picture. *Am J Surg Pathol* 11 (suppl 1):47–60, 1987.

Duray PH: Histopathology of clinical phases of human Lyme disease. *Rheum Dis Clin North Am* 15: 691–710, 1989.

Jaulhac B, Chary-Valckenaere I, Sibilia J, et al: Detection of *Borrelia burgdorferi* by DNA amplification in synovial tissue samples. *Arthritis Rheum* 39: 736–745, 1996.

Logigian EL, Kaplan RF, Steere AC: Chronic neurologic manifestations of Lyme disease. *N Engl J Med* 323: 1438–1444, 1990.

Luft BJ, Steinman CR, Neimark HC, et al: Invasion of the central nervous system by *Borrelia burgdorferi* in acute disseminated infection. *JAMA* 267:1364–1367, 1992.

Malane MS, Grant-Kels JM, Feder HM: Diagnosis of Lyme disease based on dermatologic manifestations. *Ann Intern Med* 114:490–498, 1991.

Marcus LC, Steere AC, Duray PH, et al: Fatal pancarditis in a patient with coexistent Lyme disease and babesiosis: Demonstration of spirochetes in the myocardium. *Ann Inter Med* 103:374–376, 1985.

McAlister HF, Klementowicz PT, Andrews C, et al: Lyme carditis: An important cause of reversible heart block. *Ann Intern Med* 110:339–345, 1989.

Olson JC, Esterly NB: Urticarial vasculitis and Lyme disease. *J Am Acad Dermatol* 22(supp 1):1114–1115, 1990.

Olson LJ, Okafor EC, Clements IP: Cardiac involvement in Lyme disease: Manifestations and management. *Mayo Clin Proc* 61:745–749, 1986.

Rahn DW: Lyme disease: Clinical manifestations, diagnosis, and treatment. *Semin Arthritis Rheum* 20: 201–218, 1991.

Rahn DW, Malawista SE: Lyme disease: Recommendations for diagnosis and treatment. *Ann Intern Med* 114:472–481, 1991.

Schmid GP: The global distribution of Lyme disease. *Rev Inf Dis* 7:41–50, 1985.

Sigal LH (ed): National clinical conference on Lyme disease. *Am J Med* 98(4A):1S–84S, 1995.

Sigal LH: Pseudo-Lyme disease. *Bull Rheum Dis* 44(8): 1–7, 1995.

Stanek G, Klein J, Bittner R, Glogar D: Isolation of *Borrelia burgdorferi* from myocardium of a patient with longstanding cardiomyopathy. *N Engl J Med* 322: 249–252, 1990.

Steere AC: Lyme disease. *N Engl J Med* 321:586–596, 1989.

Steere AC, Batsford WP, Weinberg M, et al: Lyme carditis: Cardiac abnormalities of Lyme disease. *Ann Intern Med* 93 (part 1):8–16, 1980.

White DJ, Chang HG, Benach JL, et al: The geographic spread and temporal increase of the Lyme disease epidemic. *JAMA* 266:1230–1236, 1991.

Zimmer G, Schaible UE, Kramer MD, et al: Lyme carditis in immunodeficient mice during experimental infection of *Borrelia burgdorferi*. *Virchows Arch Pathol Anat* 417:129–135, 1990.

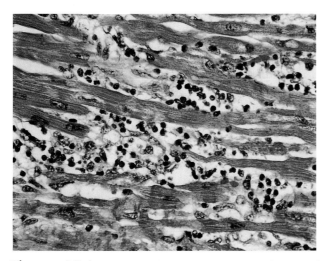

Figure 18.1. Lymphoplasmacytic myocarditis with isolated myocyte necrosis in endomyocardial biopsy of a Lyme disease patient with acute-onset unexplained heart failure.

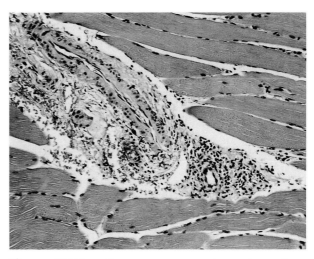

Figure 18.2. Inflammatory myopathy with small vessel vasculitis in muscle biopsy of Lyme disease patient with severe calf muscle pain.

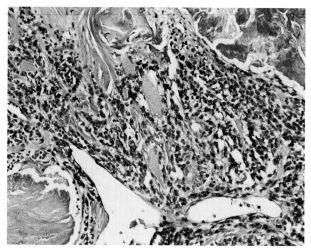

Figure 18.3. Lymphoplasmacytic synovitis in synovial biopsy of a Lyme disease patient with pain and mild effusion in a knee joint.

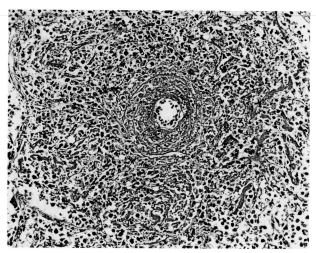

Figure 18.4. Small vessel necrotizing vasculitis as an unexpected finding in an inguinal lymph node biopsy of a Lyme disease patient with painful lymphadenopathy.

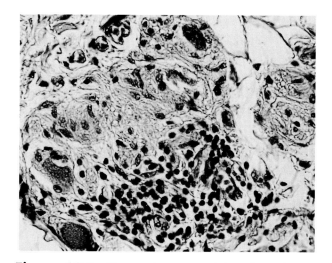

Figure 18.5. Biopsy documented lymphocytic ganglioneuritis in a Lyme disease patient with a nonspecific sensorimotor peripheral neuropathy.

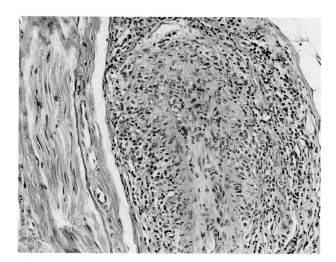

Figure 18.6. Biopsy documented polyarteritis type vasculitis in a Lyme disease patient with mononeuritis multiplex.

19. Sarcoidosis

HISTOPATHOLOGIC DEFINITION AND CLINICAL DIAGNOSIS

There is no general agreement on the definition of sarcoidosis. An international conference in 1960 rejected the morphologic definition of "a non-caseating granulomatous disease with the characteristic appearance of epithelioid tubercles with little or no necrosis" on the ground that this appearance is not pathognomonic and, instead, suggested 'a short descriptive paragraph' of the disease in place of a definition.

Sarcoidosis is a systemic, chronic, granulomatous disease of unknown etiology, affecting principally young adults 20 to 40 years of age, and presenting commonly with hilar lymphadenopathy, pulmonary infiltration, and ocular and skin lesions. However, sarcoidosis can involve virtually any organ system and thereby mimic other rheumatic diseases capable of causing fever, arthritis, uveitis, myositis, and rash, as summarized in Table 19.1.

Immunologically, sarcoidosis is a lymphoproliferative disorder in which there is depression of delayed-type hypersensitivity, imbalance of OKT4:T8 subsets (0.8/1 in sarcoidosis versus 1.8/1 in normals), hyperactive B cells, and the presence of circulating immune complexes. Activated humoral immunity in sarcoidosis is manifested by serologic evidence of polyclonal gammopathy and autoantibody production; approximately 20 to 30% of patients have tested positively for rheumatoid factor or antinuclear antibodies. Laboratory markers of disease activity include elevated serum angiotensin-converting enzyme levels, abnormal calcium metabolism, a positive Kveim-Siltzabach skin test, intrathoracic uptake of radioactive gallium, and abnormal fluorescein angiography.

The diagnosis of sarcoidosis is established most securely when the well-recognized characteristic clinicoradiologic findings are supported by histologic evidence of widespread epithelioid granulomas in multiple sites. The clinical course and prognosis correlate with the mode of onset. An acute onset usually signifies a self-limiting course often with spontaneous resolution, whereas an insidious onset may herald a chronic debilitating disease to be followed by relentless progressive fibrosis. In postmortem studies, the cause of death can be attributed to sarcoidosis and its complications in 50% of the patients.

BIOPSY DIAGNOSIS IN SARCOIDOSIS: EXTRACARDIAC INVOLVEMENTS

Non-caseating granulomas are widely disseminated in sarcoidosis. The estimated percents of patients with clinically apparent organ-involvement are: lymph nodes, 85%; lung, 85%; liver, 60%; spleen, 60%; heart, 30%;

Table 19.1 Rheumatic Manifestations of Sarcoidosis*

Manifestation	Frequency	Differential Diagnosis
Arthritis	15%	Rheumatoid arthritis; rheumatic fever; SLE; gouty arthritis; gonococcal arthritis; spondyloarthropathies
Uveitis	20%	Wegener's granulomatosis
Anterior	15%	Spondyloarthropathies
Posterior	5%	Behçet's disease
Keratoconjunctivitis	5%	Sjögren's syndrome
Proptosis	1%	Wegener's granulomatosis
Parotid gland enlargement	5%	Sjögren's syndrome
Upper airway disease (sinusitis, laryngitis, saddle nose deformity)	5%	Wegener's granulomatosis
Inflammatory myositis	5%	Dermatopolymyositis
Mononeuritis multiplex	3%	Systemic vasculitis
Facial nerve palsy	2%	Lyme disease

*Modified from Hellmann DB: Sarcoidosis. In Schumacher HR, Klippel JH, Koopman WJ (eds): *Primer on the Rheumatic Diseases, ed 10.* Atlanta, The Arthritis Foundation, 1993: 204–206.

skin, 25%; joints, 20%; kidney, 15%; bone marrow, 15%; eyes, 10%; extrapulmonary blood vessels, 10%; muscles or nerves, 5%; parotid glands or pancreas, 5%; and the central nervous system, <5%.

Biopsies serve a dual purpose in the diagnosis of sarcoidosis: to confirm the characteristic morphologic lesions and to document the unsuspected sites of involvement where the tissue samples are accessible. Extracardiac involvements in sarcoidosis that are often clinically suggestive, accessible for biopsy confirmation, and histologically show typical noncaseating granulomatous lesions include: lymph node (Fig.19.1); lung (Fig. 19.2); liver (Fig. 19.3); synovium (Fig. 19.4); skeletal muscle (Fig. 19.5); peripheral nerve (Fig. 19.6); salivary gland (Fig. 19.7) and the kidney (Fig. 19.8). Pulmonary sarcoid angiitis, originally described as pulmonary necrotizing sarcoid granulomatosis, may be seen in 30 to 50% of open lung biopsies (Fig. 19.9). Sarcoidosis of the central nervous system can occur early in the course of the disease and, occasionally, may be the presenting manifestation with pleocytosis and elevated protein as abnormal spinal fluid findings, but a brain biopsy is rarely undertaken.

BIOPSY DIAGNOSIS IN SARCOIDOSIS: CARDIAC INVOLVEMENT

Cardiac involvement in sarcoidosis has been reported to occur in up to one-third of autopsy patients but is notoriously difficult to diagnose clinically; it may remain occult even when extensive and may manifest as unexpected sudden death. The diagnosis of cardiac sarcoidosis should be considered in any young patient with arrhythmias, heart blocks, or unexplained heart failure. Sarcoid infiltration in the heart is one of the few possible causes of regional left ventricular dysfunction in the absence of significant disease of the major coronary arteries. The distribution is typically focal in the basal half of the left ventricular free wall and diffuse in the ventricular septum (Fig. 19.10), corresponding to regional akinesis and the eventual aneurysmal changes of the affected ventricle. Mitral stenosis or insufficiency from sarcoid infiltration of one or both of the valve leaflets has also been observed in specimens obtained at valve replacement surgery (Fig. 19.11); as has the diagnosis of sarcoid angiitis in samples obtained at coronary artery surgery (Fig. 19.12), and of sarcoid aortitis in surgical repair of aortic aneurysm (Fig. 19.13).

The advent of endomyocardial biopsy has greatly facilitated the antemortem diagnosis of cardiac sarcoidosis, but an isolated negative biopsy cannot always rule out the disease. Positive biopsies may have diverse appearances depending on the chronologic age and focal variations of the disease. The histopathologic spectrum of cardiac sarcoidosis in biopsies includes mild focal lymphocytic myocarditis (Fig. 19.14); extensive lymphocytic myocarditis with minimal fibrosis and without the giant cells (Fig. 19.15); focal lymphocytic myocarditis with the hint of a poorly formed giant cell in the infiltrate (Fig. 19.16); granulomatous myocarditis with giant cells and interstitial fibrosis (Fig. 19.17); extensive regional fibrosis with residual lymphocytic infiltrate (Fig. 19.18); and intramyocardial small-vessel granulomatous angiitis (Fig. 19.19). Sarcoid infiltration of the conduction system (Fig. 19.20) is a common finding in sudden death.

BIBLIOGRAPHY

Carrington CB, Gaensler EA, Mikus JP, et al: Structure and function in sarcoidosis. *Ann NY Acad Sci* 278: 265–282, 1976.

Chittock DR, Joseph MG, Paterson NAM, McFadden RG: Necrotizing sarcoid granulomatosis with pleural involvement: Clinical and radiographic features. *Chest* 106:672–676, 1994.

Churg A, Carrington CB, Gupta R: Necrotizing sarcoid granulomatosis. *Chest* 76:406–413, 1979.

Fleming HA: Cardiac sarcoidosis. *Semin Respir Med* 8: 65–71, 1986.

Flint K, Johnson N: Intrathoracic sarcoidosis. *Semin Respir Med* 8:41–51, 1986.

Fitchett DH, Oakley CM: Granulomatous mitral valve obstruction. *Br Heart J* 38:112–116, 1976.

Gedalia A, Shetty AK, Ward K, et al: Abdominal aortic aneurysm associated with childhood sarcoidosis. *J Rheumatol* 23:757–759, 1996.

Gibbs AR, Jones Williams W: The pathology of sarcoidosis. *Semin Respir Med* 8:10–16, 1986.

Graham E: Ocular sarcoidosis. *Semin Respir Med* 8: 59–64, 1986.

Hellmann DB: Sarcoidosis. In Schumacher HR, Klippel JH, Koopman WJ (eds): *Primer on the Rheumatic Diseases*, ed 10. Atlanta, The Arthritis Foundation, 1993: 204–206.

Hellman DB, Stobo JD: Sarcoidosis. In Cohen AS, Bennett JD (eds): *Rheumatology and Immunology,* ed 2. Orlando, Grune & Stratton, 1986:301–309.

Hsu RM, Connors AF, Tomashefski JF: Histologic, microbiologic, and clinical correlates of the diagnosis of sarcoidosis by transbronchial biopsy. *Arch Pathol Lab Med* 120:364–368, 1996.

James DG: Definition and classification of granulomatous disorders. *Semin Respir Med* 8:10–16, 1986.

James DG, Jones Williams W: Sarcoidosis and Other Granulomatous disorders. In Smith AH (ed): *Major Problems in Internal Medicine,* Vol 24. Philadelphia, W B Saunders, 1985.

King BP, Esparza AR, Kahn SI, Garella S: Sarcoid granulomatous nephritis: Occurring as isolated renal failure. *Arch Intern Med* 136:241–245, 1976.

Klech H: Sarcoidosis: differential diagnosis. *Semin Respir Med* 8:72–94, 1986.

Koss MN, Hochholzer L, Feigin DS, et al: Necrotizing sarcoid-like granulomatosis: Clinical, pathologic, and immunopathologic findings. *Hum Pathol* 11 (suppl): 510–519, 1980.

Lemery R, McGoon MD, Edwards WD: Cardiac sarcoidosis: A potentially treatable form of myocarditis. *Mayo Clin Proc* 60:549–554, 1985.

Lie JT: Classification of pulmonary angiitis and granulomatosis: Histopathologic perspectives. *Semin Respir Med* 10:111–121, 1989.

Lie JT, Hunt D, Valentine PA: Sudden death from cardiac sarcoidosis with involvement of conduction system. *Am J Med Sci* 267:123–128, 1974.

Matsui Y, Iwai K, Tachibana T, et al: Clinicopathological study on fatal myocardial sarcoidosis. *Ann NY Acad Sci* 278:455–469, 1976.

Mikami R, Sekiguchi M, Ryuzin Y, et al: Changes in the peripheral vasculature of various organs in patients with sarcoidosis: Possible role of microangiopathy. *Heart Vessels* 2:129–139, 1986.

Mitchell DN, Scadding JG, Heard BE, Hinson KFW: Sarcoidosis: Histopathological definition and clinical diagnosis. *J Clin Pathol* 30:395–408, 1977.

Neville E: Upper respiratory tract sarcoidosis. *Semin Respir Med* 8:52–58, 1986.

Rizzato G: Markers of activity in sarcoidosis. *Semin Respir Med* 8:30–40, 1986.

Roberts WC, McAllister HA Jr, Ferrans VJ: Sarcoidosis of the heart: A clinicopathologic study of 35 necropsy patients and review of 78 previously described necropsy patients. *Am J Med* 63:86–108, 1977.

Rosen Y, Moon S, Huang CT, et al: Granulomatous pulmonary angiitis in sarcoidosis. *Arch Pathol Lab Med* 101:170–174, 1977.

Sekiguchi M, Numao Y, Imai M, et al: Clinical and histopathological profile of sarcoidosis of the heart and acute idiopathic myocarditis: Concept through a study employing endomyocardial biopsy. I: Sarcoidosis. *Jap Circ J* 44:249–263, 1980.

Sekiguchi M, Hiroe M, Take M, et al: Clinical and histopathological profile of sarcoidosis of the heart and acute idiopathic myocarditis: Concepts through a study employing endomyocardial biopsy. II. Myocarditis. *Jap Circ J* 44:264–273, 1980.

Seminzato G: The immunology of sarcoidosis. *Semin Respir Med* 8:17–29, 1986.

Sharma OP, Kadakia D: Etiology of sarcoidosis. *Semin Respir Med* 8:95–102, 1986.

Sharma OP, Maheshwari A, Thaker K: Myocardial sarcoidosis. *Chest* 103:253–258, 1993.

Silverman KJ, Hutchins GM, Bulkley BH: Cardiac sarcoid: A clinicopathologic study of 84 unselected patients with systemic sarcoidosis. *Circulation* 58:1204–1211, 1978.

Takemura T, Matsui Y, Saiki S, Mikami R: Pulmonary vascular involvement in sarcoidosis: A report of 40 autopsy cases. *Hum Pathol* 23:1216–1223, 1992.

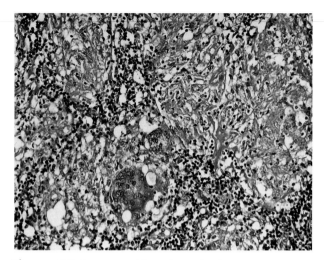

Figure 19.1. Sarcoid lymph node showing many discrete and confluent noncaseating granulomas.

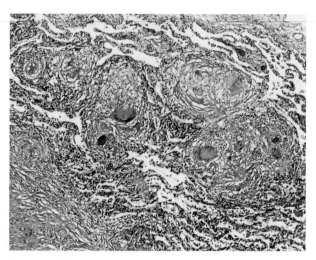

Figure 19.2. Open lung biopsy showing parenchymal noncaseating sarcoid granulomas.

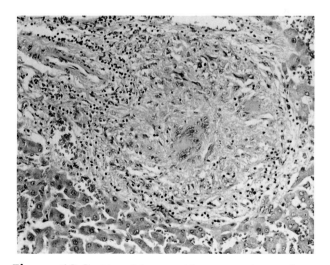

Figure 19.3. Liver biopsy with a sarcoid granuloma in the portal tract.

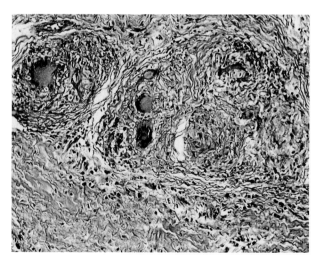

Figure 19.4. Synovial biopsy showing sarcoid granulomas and associated fibrosis.

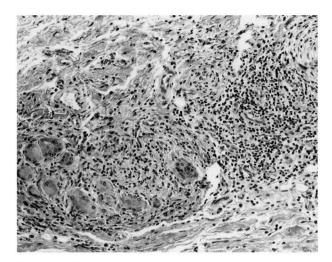

Figure 19.5. Muscle biopsy showing a granulomatous myositis in sarcoidosis.

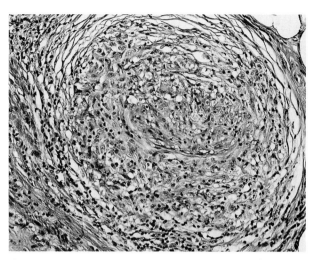

Figure 19.6. Sural nerve biopsy showing a granulomatous vasculitis of sarcoidosis.

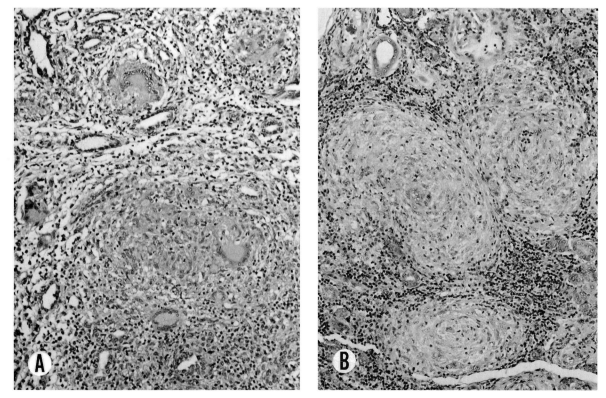

Figure 19.7. Parotid gland biopsy showing noncaseating granulomas **(A)** and small-vessel granulomatous vasculitis **(B)** in sarcoidosis.

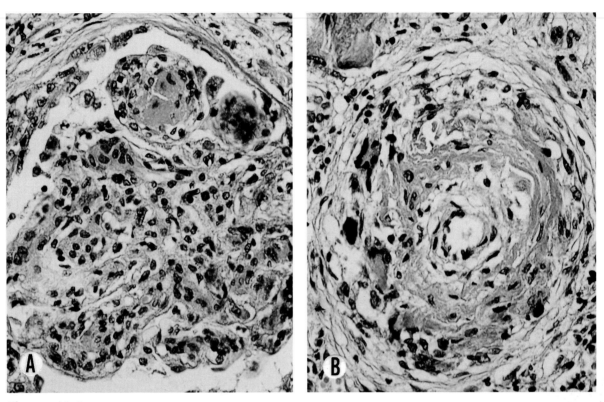

Figure 19.8. Renal biopsy showing granulomatous glomerulonephritis **(A)** and small-vessel granulomatous angiitis **(B)** in sarcoidosis.

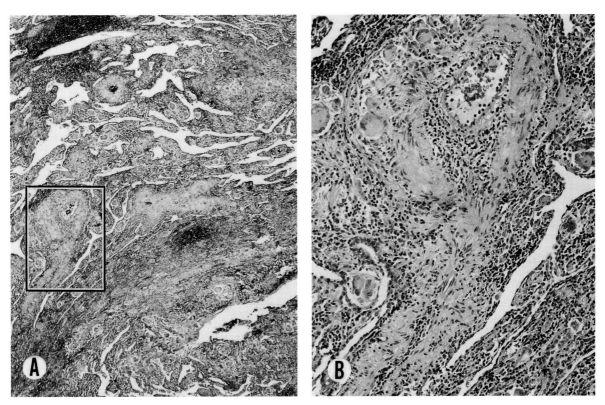

Figure 19.9. Open lung biopsy with pulmonary necrotizing sarcoid granulomatosis **(A)** and close-up view **(B)** of the framed selected example of sarcoid angiitis.

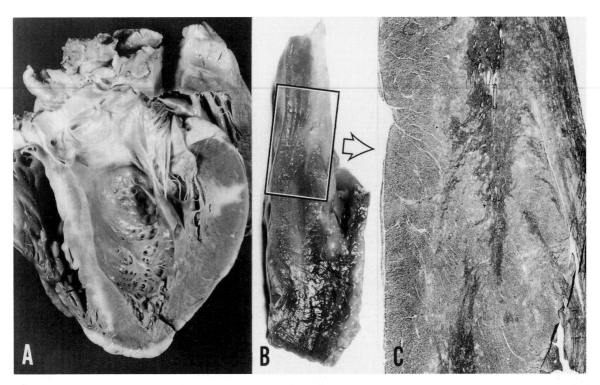

Figure 19.10. A. Characteristic appearance of sarcoid infiltration in the basal half of the left ventricular free wall as a discrete white scar and the diffuse involvement of ventricular septum. **B.** Actual thickness of the ventricular septum in profile, and the framed portion with scarring is shown as a scanning view low-magnification photomicrograph in **C** with the darker staining fibrotic areas.

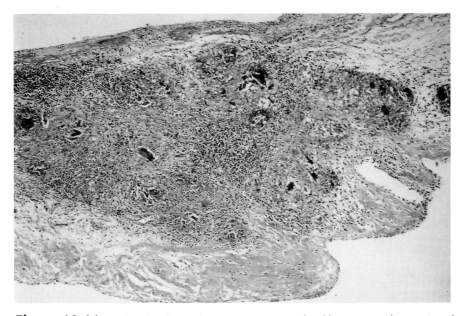

Figure 19.11. Valve leaflet with extensive sarcoid infiltration and associated fibrosis excised at valve replacement for mitral insufficiency.

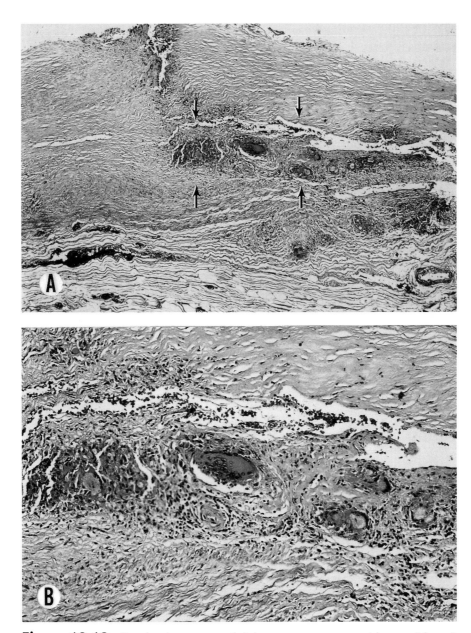

Figure 19.12. Proximal segment of right coronary artery with sarcoid angiitis (**A**) excised at surgery for interposition vein graft to relieve obstruction in a 34-year-old man, and close-up view (**B**) of the arterial wall granulomatous inflammation indicated by arrows in **A**.

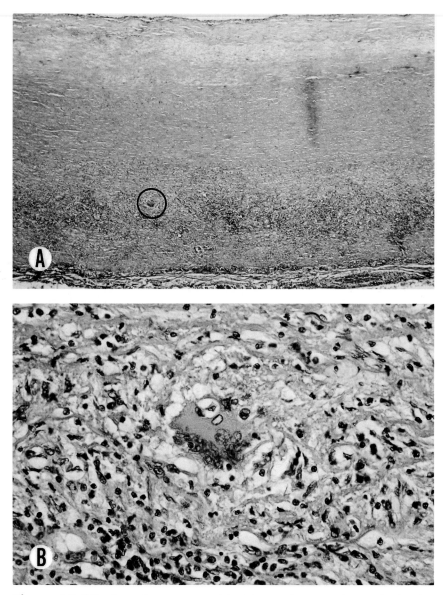

Figure 19.13. Granulomatous aortitis **(A)** seen in a specimen obtained at surgical repair of aortic aneurysm in sarcoidosis, and close-up view **(B)** of the giant cell circled in **A.**

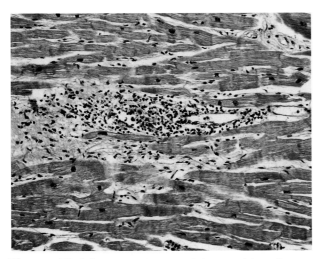

Figure 19.14. A small isolated focus of lymphocytic myocarditis in cardiac sarcoidosis.

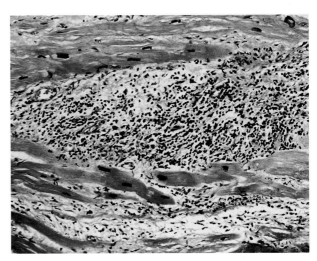

Figure 19.15. Extensive lymphocytic myocarditis with minimal fibrosis in cardiac sarcoidosis.

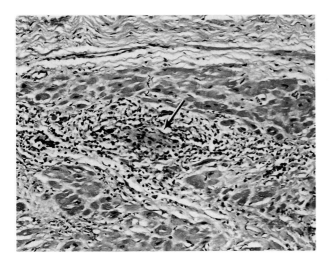

Figure 19.16. Focal lymphocytic myocarditis with an ill-formed giant cell (*arrow*) at the center of inflammatory infiltrate in cardiac sarcoidosis.

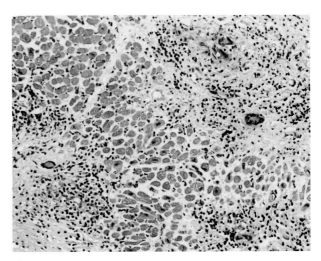

Figure 19.17. Unequivocal granulomatous myocarditis with giant cells and interstitial fibrosis in cardiac sarcoidosis.

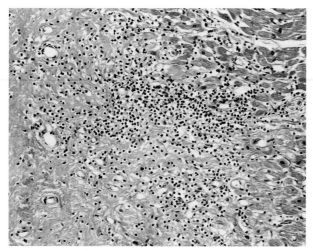

Figure 19.18. Endomyocardial biopsy in cardiac sarcoidosis showing only extensive fibrosis with residual lymphocytic infiltrate.

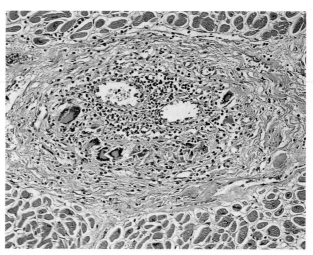

Figure 19.19. Intramyocardial small-vessel granulomatous angiitis in cardiac sarcoidosis.

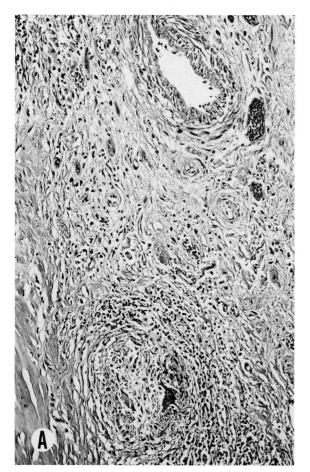

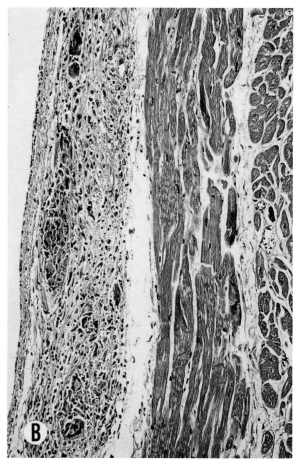

Figure 19.20. Involvement of the conduction system in sudden death from cardiac sarcoidosis, with noncaseating granulomas replacing the atrioventricular node (**A**) and the proximal segment of the left bundle branch (**B**).

20. Vasculitis Look-Alikes and the Pseudovasculitis Syndromes

WHAT ARE VASCULITIS LOOK-ALIKES?

Systemic and isolated vasculitides are a heterogeneous group of disorders, and they represent the prototypic and most important type of inflammatory rheumatic disease in clinical medicine. The manifestations of vasculitis are characteristically diverse and often unpredictable. In the absence of pathognomonic signs and symptoms or laboratory tests, the diagnosis of vasculitis is based usually on pattern recognition of the presenting clinical features, angiographic abnormalities and, where possible, biopsy findings in the affected tissues and organs. [*See* Chapter 9]

A variety of common and uncommon nonvasculitic conditions may mimic vasculitis, either clinically, angiographically, or even histologically. These are the *vasculitis look-alikes and pseudovasculitis syndromes.* The vasculitis associated with malignancy as a paraneoplastic syndrome is true vasculitis and not a vasculitis look-alike. The concept of incorporating the vasculitis look-alikes in the classification of vasculitis was first introduced a decade ago with a small selection of only six entities (Lie 1987) and the number of such entities has more than tripled now 10 years later (Table 20.1).

In clinical practice, it is imperative that the vasculitis look-alikes be distinguished from true vasculitis in order to avoid the unnecessary treatment of patients with immunosuppressive and cytotoxic agents, all of which have serious side-effects; although they are life-saving drugs for many different types of systemic vasculitis. Selected examples of the more important vasculitis look-alikes and pseudovasculitic syndromes are reviewed and the pertinent biopsy findings illustrated in this Chapter; they are described in the reverse order of frequencies, beginning with the less common large-vessel lesions to be followed by the more common small-vessel lesions.

EHLERS-DANLOS SYNDROME

Ehlers-Danlos syndrome (EDS) is a heritable disorder of collagens, and at least 11 subgroups have been identified with different clinical manifestations, biochemical defects, and inheritance patterns. The essential clinical features of EDS consist of cutaneous hyperextensibility, easy ecchymosis, and blood vessel wall fragility. Cardiovascular abnormalities have been described in type I (gravis form), type III (benign familial hypermobility syndrome), and type IV (arterial form) EDS. Vascular lesions of EDS most commonly present as single or multiple aneurysms, and arterial dissection or perforation; involvement of as many as 12 arteries in a patient has been described. Such lesions may be confused with angiitis in a variety of ways, ranging from lung microvascular injury with fatal hemoptysis mimicking pulmonary capillaritis-associated diffuse alveolar hemorrhage to angiographic simulation of multiple vasculitic aneurysms (Fig. 20.1).

NEUROFIBROMATOSIS

Neurofibromatoses comprise two clinical variants of autosomal dominant hamartomatous disorder of the neural crest with a population incidence of approximately 1:3,000 in the United States, 50% of the cases are inherited and 50% result from spontaneous mutations. Neurofibromatosis type 1 (von Recklinghausen

Table 20.1 Vasculitis Look-Alikes and Pseudovasculitis Syndromes

- Hypertensive vascular disease
- Arterial dysplasia, hypoplasia, or coarctation
- Vaso-occlusive disease of antiphospholipid syndromes
- Cholesterol atheroembolism
- Cardiac myxoma embolism
- Endocarditis thromboembolism
- Chronic ergotism
- Blackfoot disease (environmental chronic arsenism)
- Radiation arteriopathy
- Post-rubella syndrome
- Neurofibromatosis
- Ehlers-Danlos syndrome
- Pseudoxanthoma elasticum
- Inflammatory aneurysm
- Inflammatory pseudotumor
- Köhlmeier-Dagos disease (malignant atrophic papulosis)
- Sweet's syndrome (acute febrile neutrophilic dermatosis)
- Intravascular lymphomatosis (malignant angioendotheliomatosis)
- Leptomeningeal dissemination of malignant glioma
- Pheochromocytoma, paraganglioma

disease, or the classic form), identified with a gene located on chromosome 17, is characterized by multiple *café au lait* spots, cutaneous neurofibromas, Lisch nodules (pigmented iris hamartomas), axillary freckling, learning disabilities, and a variety of skeletal, endocrine, neoplastic, and other clinical manifestations. Neurofibromatosis type 2 (acoustic or central form of neurofibromatosis), identified with a gene located on chromosome 22, is characterized by acoustic neuromas and other neural tumors such as meningiomas, gliomas, and schwannomas.

Vascular lesions are associated with neurofibromatosis type 1, the exact frequency has not been determined but is probably close to 10% of the patients. Both proliferative and aneurysmal arterial lesions have been observed; the former is more common, involving chiefly the renal arteries causing renovascular hypertension, and less frequently other visceral and peripheral arteries, or rarely the aorta as abdominal coarctation. The proliferative vascular lesions of neurofibromatosis may occur alone or alternate with aneurysmal disease, mimicking vasculitis angiographically or even histologically with cursory examination (Fig. 20.2).

ARTERIAL FIBROMUSCULAR DYSPLASIA

Arterial fibromuscular dysplasia (FMD) is considered to be a developmental anomaly of small and medium-sized arteries, and rarely veins, in which the vessel wall is altered by dysplasia, hypoplasia, and/or hyperplasia of its normal fibromuscular components resulting in alternating stenosis and aneurysmal dilation of the lumen. Four morphologic subtypes of FMD have been identified: medial FMD (90–95%), intimal fibroplasia (2–3%), adventitial fibroplasia (2–3%), and mediolytic dysplasia (2–3%). FMD occurs most commonly in the renal arteries of young women as a common cause of renovascular hypertension; followed in descending order of frequencies, the internal carotid arteries and visceral arteries, and only very rarely the coronary arteries. The association of FMD with intracranial berry aneurysms occurs more often than by chance.

Vaso-occlusive disease and/or intramural arterial dissection are the clinically significant complications of FMD. Renal artery FMD with medial dissection and microaneurysms has often been misdiagnosed angiographically as polyarteritis nodosa (Fig. 20.3), as has other visceral artery FMD. There have been a number of such cases of FMD with presumptive diagnosis of vas-

culitis, unsubstantiated by histologic confirmation, for which the patients received corticosteroids and/or cytotoxic agents with tragic outcome. The misguided drug therapy with immuno-suppressive agents not only has no beneficial effects on the FMD but it also may have hastened the patient's demise from sepsis and the uncorrected complications of FMD.

CHRONIC ERGOTISM

Medieval epidemics of ergotism caused by eating bread and cereal made from rye contaminated by the fungus *Claviceps purpurea* was documented in 1670 and called 'St. Anthony's fire' in reference to the blackened gangrenous limb believed consumed by the 'holy fire'. Even today, chronic ergotism-induced vasospastic arterial disease should be remembered as a possible cause of peripheral, visceral, or coronary ischemia from prolonged use of ergotamine tartrate preparations for migraine. To the unwary, angiographic findings of chronic ergotism-induced vasculopathy may be mistaken as vasculitis (Fig. 20.4). Again, the correct treatment is to discontinue the use of ergot compounds and not immunosuppressive therapy.

HYPERTENSIVE VASCULAR DISEASE

A classic example of pseudovasculitic syndrome is the small-vessel disease in severe, sustained systemic or pulmonary hypertension. In renal biopsies, the kidney in malignant hypertension often shows arteriolar fibrinoid necrosis and necrotizing vasculitis of small arteries (Fig. 20.5A). The same morphologic type of vascular injury also occurs in the mesenteric circulation with sudden rise of the perfusion pressure, say, after surgical repair of coarctation of the aorta. Similarly, the small-vessel necrotizing vasculitis in a lung biopsy (Fig. 20.5B) signifies the most severe form (Heath-Edwards grade 6) of plexogenic pulmonary hypertension. The distinction of hypertensive vascular disease from true vasculitis is usually not a diagnostic problem when one does not overlook the obviously characteristic clinical settings in systemic and pulmonary hypertension when interpreting the biopsies.

Occasionally, arterial spasm from acute elevation of the blood pressure, say, in pregnancy or postpartum, may produce cerebral angiographic changes closely mimicking angiitis of the central nervous system. Such vasospastic changes are reversible with normalization of blood pressure, and also not associated with other evidence of true cerebral vasculitis.

CARDIAC MYXOMA EMBOLISM

Cardiac myxoma embolism often mimics vasculitis either as multiple arterial microaneurysms (Fig. 20.6) or small-vessel occlusive disease, and the correct diagnosis cannot be made without critical evaluation of a biopsy (Figs. 20.7 and 20.8). Arterial aneurysms are an angiographic hallmark of polyarteritis nodosa, but other vasculitic and nonvasculitic conditions, including cardiac myxoma embolism, may also be associated with angiographically demonstrable arterial microaneurysms. Cardiac myxoma is the only tumor known to cause aneurysmal formation with embolization; these peculiar aneurysms have been observed in systemic and cerebral circulation, and also in pulmonary vasculature with cardiac myxomas arising from the right-sided chambers of the heart. Embolized cardiac myxomas are apparently autonomous and capable of aneurysmal formation following surgical resection of the primary tumor in the heart.

INTRAVASCULAR LYMPHOMATOSIS

Also known as 'malignant angioendotheliomatosis' or 'angiocentric lymphoma', intravascular lymphomatosis (IVL) is an uncommon and usually lethal disease characterized by the peculiar systemic intravascular proliferation of neoplastic lymphoid cells, and frequently involving the cutaneous, visceral, pulmonary, and cerebral vasculature. IVL in all different sites may mimic vasculitis. Cerebral IVL cannot be easily distinguished from the equally high-mortality primary angiitis of the central nervous system either clinically or angiographically; a clinician often has no choice but to resort to a brain biopsy for confirmation of diagnosis (Figs. 20.9 and 20.10).

CHOLESTEROL ATHEROEMBOLISM

Cholesterol atheromatous embolism (CAE) is the most common form of vasculitis look-alike known in medicine; it surpasses all other imitators by its sheer number and the seemingly unlimited variety of clinical presentations (Table 20.2). Spontaneous CAE has been detected in 3 to 9% of unselected autopsy populations,

Table 20.2. Clinical Manifestations of Systemic Cholesterol Atheroembolism*

Skin and Extremities	*Neuro-Ophthalmologic*
Livido reticularis	Transient ischemic attacks
Blue or purple toe syndrome	Stroke
Digital infarcts	Encephalopathy
Gangrene	Seizure
Muscle	Amaurosis fugax
Myalgias	Asymptomatic retinal arteriole plaques
Rhabdomyolysis	Central or branch retinal artery occlusion
Elevated creatine kinase and aldolase	Homonymous hemianopia
Myoglobinuria	Ophthalmoparesis
Renal	*Bowel*
Azotemia, proteinuria and hematuria	Abdominal pain and nausea
Acute and chronic renal failure	Gastrointestinal hemorrhage
Acute-onset hypertension	Mesenteric infarction
Cardiac	*Pancreas*
Myocardial ischemia/infarction	Pancreatitis
Nonspecific Laboratory Abnormalities	Hyperglycemia
Elevated erythrocyte sedimentation rate	Elevated amylase and lipase
Elevated antinuclear antibody titer	
Leukocytosis and eosinophilia	

*Modified from Jacobson DM. *Surv Ophthalmol* 1991; 35:23–27.

and CAE is 5 to 10 times more common in patients over the age of 50 years who, during life, had undergone aortic catheterization or aortic surgery.

Historically, CAE was first described by Panum in 1862, and interest in CAE evolved slowly over the next 100 years from a pathologic curiosity to clinical entity (Moldveen-Geronimus, et al. 1967). Today, CAE remains a diagnosis that is often overlooked or not stressed by the clinician and pathologist alike. CAE may be asymptomatic, having been observed merely as an incidental autopsy or biopsy finding. When symptomatic, CAE has been dubbed 'the great masquerader' because it may be found in virtually any organ or tissue and mimic a wide variety of clinically diverse syndromes, most notably vasculitis. There are no pathognomonic laboratory tests for CAE. The correct diagnosis cannot be made without histologic documentation of embolization of the telltale spindle-shaped cholesterol crystals in various target organs, and serial sections may be necessary for a positive identification of atheroembolism.

The following selected diagnostic biopsies illustrate the diversity of clinical disorders with CAE mimicking vasculitis: renal biopsies for the unexplained renal failure with hypertension syndrome (Figs. 20.11 and 20.12); muscle biopsies in the acute lower limb ischemia-blue toe syndrome (Figs. 20.13 to 20.16); bowel resections in ischemic bowel disease (Figs. 20.17 and 20.18); laparotomy for acute pancreatitis (Fig. 20.19); cholecystectomy for acute acalculous cholecystitis (Fig. 20.20); biopsy of a tender testis (Fig. 20.21) and painful lymphadenopathy (Fig. 20. 22) to rule out vasculitis; lung biopsy to rule out pulmonary vasculitis (Fig. 20.23); and brain biopsy to rule out primary angiitis of the central nervous system (Fig. 20.24).

OTHERS

In general, any systemic disorders with multiple and variable signs and symptoms, abnormal but nonspecific laboratory test results, abnormal angiographic, ultrasound, and/or other imaging findings can be a candidate for vasculitis or a vasculitis look-alike, and the distinction cannot be made without critical evaluation of an adequate biopsy of the affected parts. Other examples of vasculitis look-alikes not illustrated here but are no less important for the patients concerned and their proper management, include: vaso-occlusive disease of

antiphospholipid syndromes; post-rubella syndrome; radiation arteriopathy; blackfoot disease (environmental chronic arsenism); endocarditis thromboembolism; pseudoxanthoma elasticum; Sweet's syndrome (acute febrile neutrophilic dermatosis); Köhlmeier-Dagos disease (malignant atrophic papulosis); inflammatory aneurysm; inflammatory pseudotumor; leptomeningeal dissemination of malignant glioma; and pheochromocytoma.

The number of new vasculitis look-alikes and pseudovasculitis syndromes will undoubtedly continue to grow as clinicians and pathologists become aware of these important masqueraders, the correct diagnosis of which will seriously influence the choice of drug treatment and plan of management.

BIBLIOGRAPHY

Anderson WR: Necrotizing angiitis associated with embolization of cholesterol. *Am J Clin Pathol* 43: 65–71, 1965.

Anderson WR, Braverman T: Colon perforation due to cholesterol embolism. *Hum Pathol* 22: 839–841, 1991.

Anderson WR, Richards AM: Evaluation of lower extremity muscle biopsies in the diagnosis of atheroembolism. *Arch Pathol Lab Med* 86: 535–541, 1968.

Blundell JW: Small bowel stricture secondary to multiple cholesterol emboli. *Histopathology* 13: 459–462, 1988.

Cappiello RA, Espinosa LR, Adelman H, et al: Cholesterol embolism: A pseudovasculitis syndrome. *Semin Arthritis Rheum* 18: 240–246, 1989.

Carnevale NJ, Delany HM: Cholesterol embolization to the cecum with bowel infarction. *Arch Surg* 106: 94–96, 1973.

Case Records of the Massachusetts General Hospital: Case 31-1995. *N Engl J Med* 333: 992–999, 1995.

Case Records of the Massachusetts General Hospital: Case 11-1996. *N Engl J Med* 334: 973–979, 1996.

Cikrit DF, Miles JH, Silver D: Spontaneous arterial perforation: The Ehlers-Danlos specter. *J Vasc Surg* 5: 248–255, 1987.

den Butler G, van Bockel JH, Aarts JCNM: Arterial

fibrodysplasia: Rapid progression complicated by rupture of a visceral aneurysm into gastrointestinal tract. *J Vasc Surg* 7: 449–453, 1988.

Faggioli GL, Gargiulo M, Bertoni F, et al: Hypertension due to an aneurysm of the left renal artery in a patient with neurofibromatosis. *Ann Vasc Surg* 6: 456–459, 1992.

Falanga V, Fine MJ, Kapoor WJ: The cutaneous manifestations of cholesterol crystal embolization. *Arch Dermatol* 122: 1194–1198, 1986.

Feinmann NL, Yakovac WC: Neurofibromatosis in childhood. *J Pediatr* 76: 339–346, 1970.

Fine MJ, Kapoor WJ, Falanga V: Cholesterol crystal embolization: A review of 221 cases in the English literature. *Angiology* 38: 769–784, 1987.

Flory CM: Arterial occlusion produced by emboli from eroded aortic atheromatous plaques. *Am J Pathol* 21: 549–565, 1945.

Francis J, Kapoor WJ: Intestinal pseudopolyps and gastrointestinal hemorrhage due to cholesterol crystal embolization. *Am J Med* 85: 269–271, 1988.

Garner BF, Burns P, Bunning RD, Laureno R: Acute blood pressure elevation can mimic angiographic appearance of cerebral vasculitis. *J Rheumatol* 17: 93–97, 1993.

Gertner E, Lie JT: Pulmonary capillaritis, alveolar hemorrhage and recurrent microvascular thrombosis in primary antiphospholipid syndrome. *J Rheumatol* 20: 1224–1228, 1993.

Glass J, Hochberg FH, Miller DC: Intravascular lymphomatosis: A systemic disease with neurologic manifestations. *Cancer* 71: 56–64, 1993.

Goldfischer JD: Acute myocardial infarction secondary to ergot therapy. *N Engl J Med* 262: 860–863, 1960.

Gore I, Collins DP: Spontaneous atheromatous embolization: Review of literature and a report. *Am J Clin Pathol* 33: 416–426, 1960.

Gore I, McCombs HL, Linquist RL: Observations on the fate of cholesterol emboli. *J Atheroscler Res* 4: 527–535, 1964.

Green FL, Ariyan S, Stansel HC Jr: Mesenteric and peripheral vascular ischemia secondary to ergotism. *Surgery* 81: 176–179, 1977.

Green JM, Longley S, Edwards NL, et al: Vasculitis associated with malignancy: Experience with 13 patients and literature review. *Medicine* 67: 222–230, 1988.

Greer KE, Cooper PH: Sweet's syndrome (acute febrile neutrophilic dermatosis). *Clin Rheum Dis* 8: 427–441, 1982.

Halper J, Factor S: Coronary lesions in neurofibromatosis associated with vasospasm and myocardial infarction. *Am Heart J* 108: 420–422, 1984.

Halpern M, Currarino G: Vascular lesion causing hypertension in neurofibromatosis. *N Engl J Med* 273: 248–251, 1965.

Herman C, Kupsky WJ, Rogers L, et al: Leptomeningeal dissemination of malignant glioma simulating cerebral vasculitis: Case report with angiographic and pathological studies. *Stroke* 26: 2366–2370, 1995.

Huffman JL, Gahtan V, Bowers VD, Mills JL: Neurofibromatosis and arterial aneurysms. *Am Surgeon* 62: 311–314, 1996.

Hunter GC, Malone JM, Moore WS, et al: Vascular manifestations in patients with Ehlers-Danlos syndrome. *Arch Surg* 117: 495–498, 1982.

Huston KA, Coombs JJ, Lie JT: Left atrial myxoma simulating peripheral vasculitis. *Mayo Clin Proc* 53: 752–756, 1978.

Jacobson DM: Systemic cholesterol microembolization syndrome masquerading as giant cell arteritis. *Surv Ophthalmol* 35: 23–27, 1991.

Janssens E, Hommel M, Mounier-Vehier F, et al: Postpartum cerebral angiopathy possibly due to bromocriptine therapy. *Stroke* 26: 128–130, 1995.

Jones DB, Iannaccone PM: Atheromatous emboli in renal biopsies: An ultrastructural study. *Am J Pathol* 78: 261–276, 1975.

Kalter DC, Rudolph A, McGavran M: Livedo reticularis due to multiple cholesterol emboli. *J Am Acad Dermatol* 13: 235–242, 1985.

Leonhardt ETG, Kullenberg KPG: Bilateral myxoma with multiple arterial aneurysms: A syndrome mimicking polyarteritis nodosa. *Am J Med* 62: 792–794, 1977.

Lie JT: Coronary vasculitis: A review in the current scheme of classification of vasculitis. *Arch Pathol Lab Med* 111: 224–233, 1987.

Lie JT: The classification and diagnosis of vasculitis in large and medium-sized blood vessels. *Pathol Ann* 22(part 2): 125–162, 1987.

Lie JT: Systemic and isolated vasculitis: A rational approach to classification and pathologic diagnosis. *Pathol Ann* 24(part 1): 25–114, 1989.

Lie JT: Vasculitis in the antiphospholipid syndrome: Thrombosis or vasculitis, or both? *J Rheumatol* 16: 713–715, 1989.

Lie JT: Cholesterol atheromatous embolism: The great masquerader revisited. *Pathol Ann* 27(part 2): 17–50, 1992.

Lie JT: Malignant angioendotheliomatosis (intravascular lymphoma) simulating primary angiitis of the central nervous system. *Arthritis Rheum* 35: 831–834, 1992.

Lie JT: Vasculitis simulators and look-alikes. *Curr Opin Rheumatol* 4: 47–55, 1992.

Lie JT: Vasculitis in the antiphospholipid syndrome: Culprit or consort? *J Rheumatol* 21: 397–399, 1994.

Lie JT: Nomenclature and classification of vasculitis: Plus ça change, plus c'est la même chose. *Arthritis Rheum* 37: 181–186, 1994.

Lie JT: Vasculitis look-alikes and pseudovasculitis syndromes. *Curr Diag Pathol* 2: 78–85, 1995.

Lie JT: Vasculitis associated with infectious agents. *Curr Opin Rheumatol* 8: 26–29, 1996.

Lüscher TF, Essendoh LK, Lie JT, et al: Renovascular hypertension: A rare cardiovascular manifestation of Ehlers-Danlos syndrome. *Mayo Clin Proc* 62: 223–229, 1987.

Lüscher TF, Lie JT, Stanson AW, et al: Arterial fibromuscular dysplasia: A review. *Mayo Clin Proc* 62: 931–952, 1987.

Magee R: Saint Anthony's Fire revisited: Vascular problems associated with migraine medication. *Med J Aust* 154: 145–149, 1991.

Mandelsohn J, Bulkley B, Hutchins G: Cardiovascular manifestations of pseudoxanthoma elasticum. *Arch Pathol Lab Med* 102: 298–302, 1978.

McColl GJ, Fraser K: Pheochromocytoma and pseudovasculitis. *J Rheumatol* 22: 1442–1443, 1995.

Meyers DS, Grim CE, Keitzer WF: Fibromuscular dysplasia of the renal artery with medial dissection: A case simulating polyarteritis nodosa. *Am J Med* 56: 412–416, 1974.

Moldveen-Geronimus M, Merriam JC Jr: Cholesterol embolism: From pathological curiosity to clinical entity. *Circulation* 35: 946–953, 1967.

Panum PL: Experimentelle Beitrage zur Lehre von der Embolie. *Virchows Arch Pathol Anat* 25: 308–310, 1862.

Pilz P, Hartjes HJ: Fibromuscular dysplasia and multiple dissecting aneurysms of intracranial arteries: A further case of moyamoya syndrome. *Stroke* 7: 393–398, 1976.

Reubi F: Neurofibromatose et lésions vascularis. *Schweiz Med Wochenschr* 75: 463–465, 1945.

Salyer WR, Salyer DC: The vascular lesions of neurofibromatosis. *Angiology* 25: 510–519, 1974.

Sánchez-Guerrero J, Gutiérrz-Urena S, Vidaller A, et al: Vasculitis as a paraneoplastic syndrome: Report of 11 cases and review of the literature. *J Rheumatol* 17: 1458–1462, 1990.

Schürch W, Messerli FH, Genest CC, et al: Arterial hypertension and neurofibromatosis: Renal artery stenosis and coarctation of abdominal aorta. *Can Med Assoc J* 113: 879–885, 1975.

Sheiner NM, Miller N, Lachance C: Arterial complications of Ehlers-Danlos syndrome. *J Cardiovasc Surg* 26: 291–296, 1985.

Su WPD, Schroeder AL, Lee DA, et al: Clinical and histologic findings in Dagos syndrome (malignant atrophic papulosis). *Cutis* 35: 131–138, 1985.

Thomas MH: Myxoma masquerading as polyarteritis nodosa. *J Rheumatol* 8: 133–137, 1981.

Travers RL, Allison DL, Brettle RP, Hughes GRN: Polyarteritis nodosa: A clinical and angiographic study. *Semin Arthritis Rheum* 8: 184–199, 1979.

Wold LE, Lie JT: Cardiac myxoma: Clinicopathologic profile, *Am J Pathol* 101: 219–240, 1980.

Yost BA, Vogelsang JP, Lie JT: Fatal hemoptysis in Ehlers-Danlos syndrome. *Chest* 107: 465–467, 1995.

Young DK, Burton MF, Herman JH: Multiple cholesterol emboli syndrome simulating systemic necrotizing vasculitis. *J Rheumatol* 13: 423–426, 1986.

Zaytsev P, Miller K, Pellettiere EV: Cutaneous cholesterol emboli with infarction clinically mimicking heparin necrosis. *Angiology* 37: 471–476, 1986.

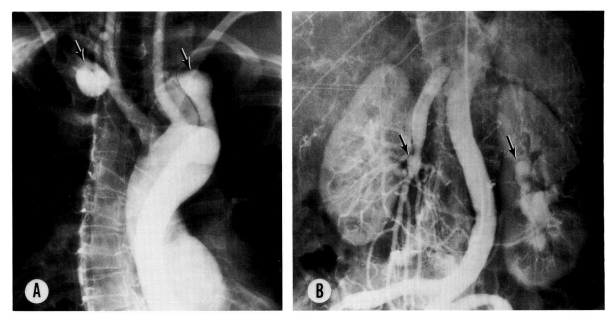

Figure 20.1. Thoracic **(A)** and abdominal **(B)** aortograms in Ehlers-Danlos syndrome showing multiple arterial aneurysms (*arrows*) mimicking systemic vasculitis.

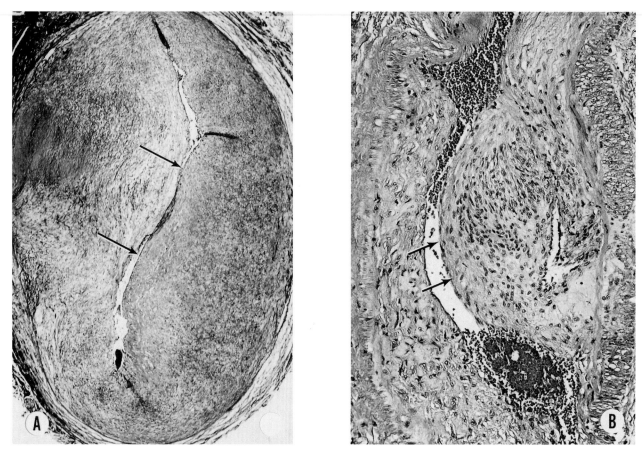

Figure 20.2. Renal artery **(A)** and mesenteric arteriole **(B)** in neurofibromatosis type 1, showing intimal prolif-erative vasculopathy with marked stenosis (*arrows*) clinically and angiographically mimicking vasculitis.

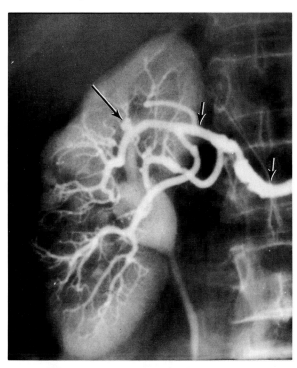

Figure 20.3. Angiogram of right renal artery fibromuscular dysplasia with irregular stenosis of the extrarenal segment (*short arrows*) and an intrarenal microaneurysm (*long arrow*) mimicking polyarteritis nodosa.

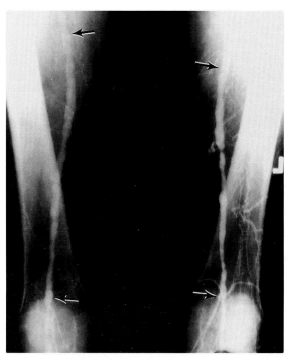

Figure 20.4. Bilateral femoral arteriograms showing irregular long and short segmental stenoses and dilations (*arrows*) in chronic ergotism mimicking vasculitis.

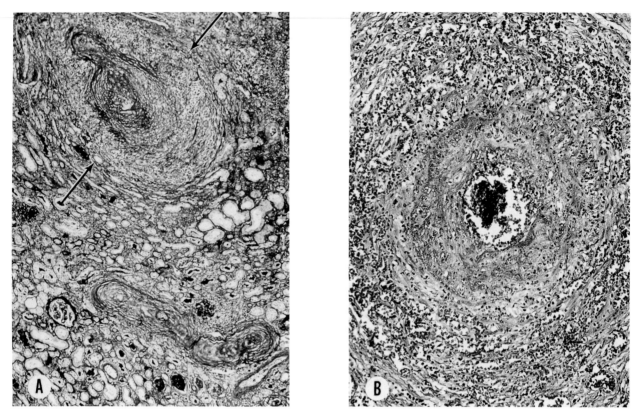

Figure 20.5. A. Necrotizing vasculitis of a small intralobar artery of the kidney in malignant hypertension. **B.** Small-vessel necrotizing vasculitis in severe (Heath-Edwards grade 6) plexogenic pulmonary hypertension.

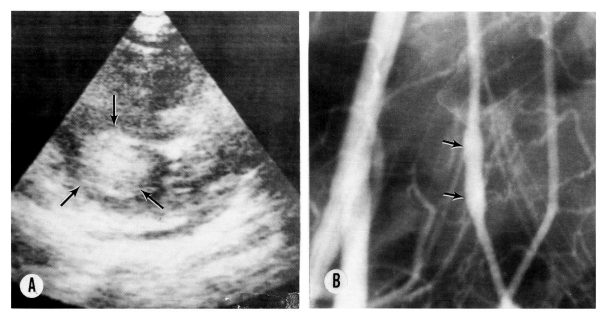

Figure 20.6. A. Two-dimensional echocardiogram demonstrating a large echo-dense left atrial myxoma (*arrows*) which was surgically resected. **B.** Right iliofemoral arteriogram of the same patient 9 months later demonstrating segmental aneurysms with stenosis in-between.

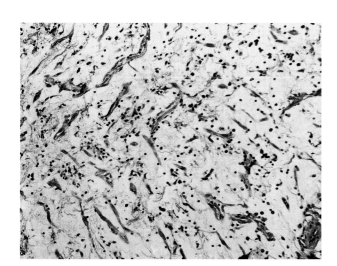

Figure 20.7. Typical histopathology of a surgically resected left atrial myxoma composed of slender tadpole-like lepidic cells.

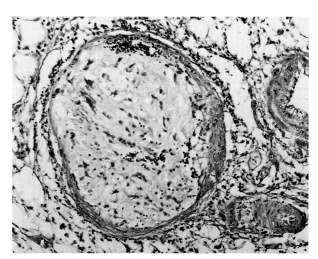

Figure 20.8. Cardiac myxoma embolus in the muscle biopsy of a patient thought to have polyarteritis in whom the myxoma illustrated in **Fig. 20.7** was subsequently resected.

208

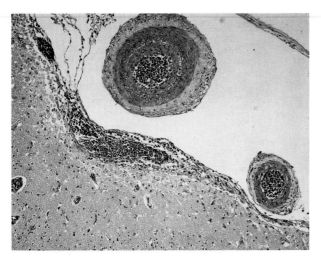

Figure 20.9. Unexpected finding of leptomeningeal intravascular lymphoma in a brain biopsy to rule out angiitis of the central nervous system.

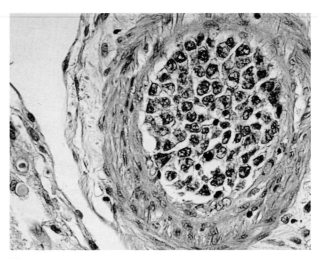

Figure 20.10. Close-up view of the large noncohesive malignant cells of intravascular lymphoma shown in **Fig. 20.9.**

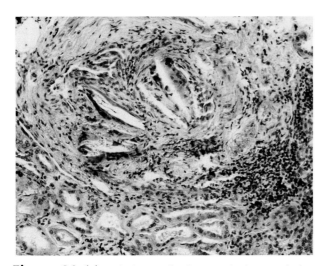

Figure 20.11. Cholesterol atheroembolus occluding an intrabolar artery in renal biopsy to rule out vasculitis of a patient with unexplained renal failure.

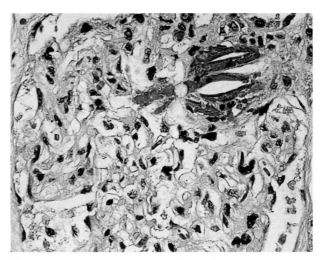

Figure 20.12. Spindle-shaped cholesterol crystals in the glomerular hilar arteriole of the same biopsy shown in **Fig. 20.11.**

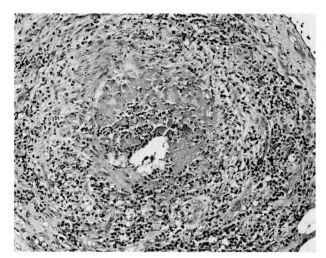

Figure 20.13. Atheroembolus with intense inflammatory infiltrate in a muscle biopsy mimicking vasculitis. Note no cholesterol crystals are seen in this section.

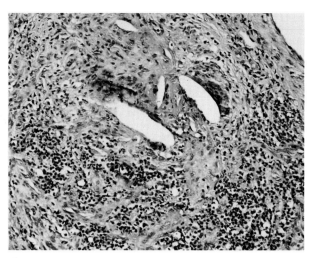

Figure 20.14. The telltale cholesterol crystals of atheroembolus seen in a subsequent serial section of the same biopsy shown in **Fig. 20.13.**

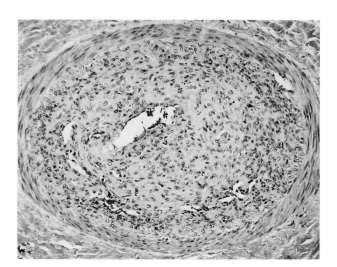

Figure 20.15. Organized old atheroembolus in a muscle biopsy with a telltale cholesterol crystal in the lumen, without it the diagnosis could not have been made.

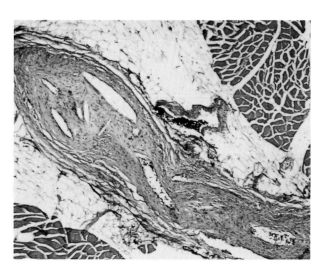

Figure 20.16. Atheroembolus in a small artery of muscle biopsy for ruling out vasculitis.

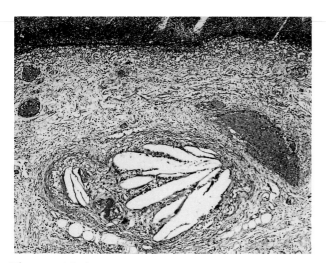

Figure 20.17. Atheroembolus in submucosal artery of colon resected for infarcted bowel.

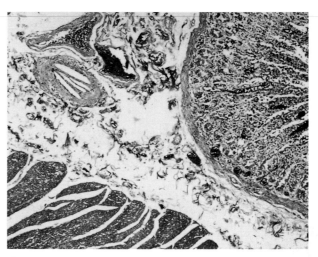

Figure 20.18. Atheroembolus in submucosal artery of jejunum resected for infarcted bowel.

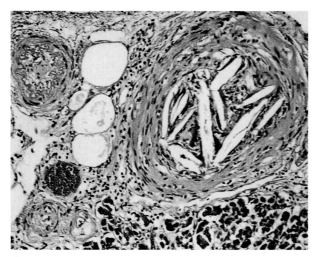

Figure 20.19. Atheroembolus in pancreatic biopsy obtained at surgery for acute pancreatitis.

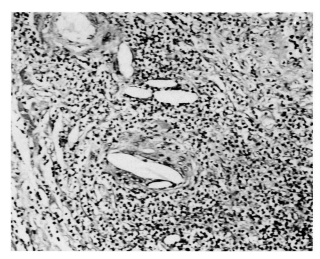

Figure 20.20. Atheroembolus found in a gallbladder removed for acalculous cholecystitis.

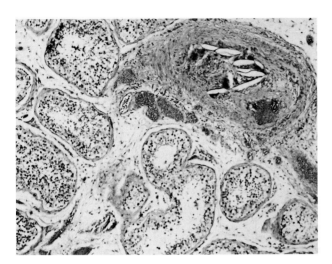

Figure 20.21. Atheroembolus seen in a testicular biopsy for ruling out polyarteritis nodosa.

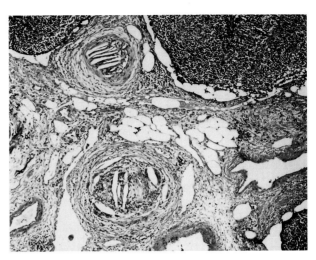

Figure 20.22. Atheroembolus found unexpectedly in biopsy for painful lymphadenopathy.

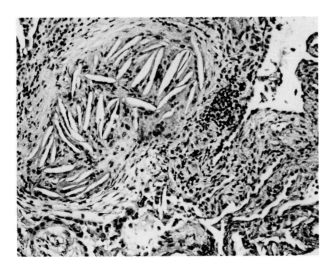

Figure 20.23. Atheroembolus in lung biopsy for ruling out pulmonary vasculitis.

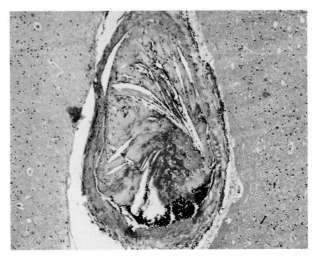

Figure 20.24. Atheroembolus in brain biopsy for ruling out cerebral angiitis.

Index